Losing our minds

Also by Patricia Worby, PhD

THE SCAR THAT WON'T HEAL 2015 REV 2018

THE WORLD WITHIN 2017

Losing our minds

A cellular view of life and healthy ageing

Engaging metabolic mechanisms for healing

By Patricia Worby, PhD

Kdp publishing

A catalogue record for this book is available from the British Library.

ISBN: 9781793103697

Imprint: Independently published through kdp

DEDICATION

To my partner Jill who has subtly supported me unconditionally in all my writing/speaking/ practice endeavours. She has put up with the endless evenings of my being online studying with (mostly) little complaint. She has also opened my eyes to the greatest inspiration of all – the natural world and all its wonders. I had always eschewed nature as being outside the important realm of study as it was just 'there'. I now appreciate how subtly and deeply we, the earth and all of life are intricately interwoven.

How to use this book

I have attempted to make this book open to all health seekers, regardless of outlook. I myself have a foot in both the scientific *and* the holistic fields. I introduce any necessary scientific information in an accessible way with plenty of illustrations and a glossary of all technical/scientific terms (all first mentions of such important concepts are in bold and briefly described in the text). But I also include practical examples of what we can *do* towards the end of each chapter because I want people to become empowered in their journey towards health. Everything is fully referenced and research-supported with a final index and reference section for those of you who want to follow up this aspect. Each chapter stands alone, although it references other chapters where necessary.

Chapters One and Two outline some key concepts of cells and the body. You may wish to skip some of the more detailed information but please do look at the diagrams – all are carefully chosen to summarise the key information. I have always attempted to make the science accessible as I believe it is so key to understanding our world. So please persevere.

Chapters Three and Four look at how we consider the world from a cellular point of view and make modifications via diet, exercise, stress, etc.

Chapters Five and Six look at disturbances to normal functioning, including the so-called 'diseases of ageing', which are usually nothing of the sort (although they are linked with ageing, they are modifiable). We can intervene to modify those processes via epigenetics and I show you how.

Chapters Seven and Eight look at two categories of disease that are both most feared and most linked with ageing; dementia and cancer. I attempt to redefine those diseases as metabolic dysfunctions and therefore neither inevitable nor incurable but, seen through the lens of cell function, modifiable or even reversible. By paying attention to early intervention/cell regenerative actions you can prevent them.

In Chapter Nine I look at a mind-body 'bigger picture' perspective of life and ageing via the influence of the mind beyond the brain.

I encourage you to delve in – either by reading in the order presented or via a pick and mix approach as each chapter can stand alone. It's up to you.
But, please can I make a request – if you've enjoyed the information presented herein **please write me an amazon review**. Thank you

TABLE OF CONTENTS:

LIST of FIGURES and TABLES

FOREWORD

We only destroy the things that we do not value and we can only value the things that we understand

Rachel Carson, author of Silent Spring

PREFACE

My aim for this (third) book is as a long culmination (and rumination) on why we are suffering an epidemic of chronic disease currently. I have already dealt with aspects of childhood trauma/unresolved emotions and the microbiome in the first and second books respectively and now it's time to turn my attention to ageing and disease – but from a cellular view.

With this more diminutive but complex perspective, we see that disease is not a natural consequence of ageing as modern medicine would have you believe. It is, in fact, a *metabolic response to the toxicity of our lives*; in the air we breathe, the food we eat, the thoughts we think and the relationships we have in this 21st century world. That we are destroying our environment with our imbalanced perspective on money and material gain as the sole focus of life, is not news to most people. But that this is being *reflected at a cellular level* with toxins clogging our inner world, is perhaps a new (but highly research-supported) area of understanding. The unprecedented (and accelerating) levels of toxic pollutants in our water and air during the last 50 years, most of which are novel to the body and therefore which it has not had time to adapt to, are destroying our inner world too. But I have an idea that with the ingenuity and resourcefulness that is also a feature of the human species, we will overcome these temporary delusions and transgressions. If we don't, we will be eliminated evolutionarily just like the dinosaurs were in their turn.

Find me on www.patriciaworby.co.uk, www.alchemytherapies.co.uk and patreon.com/patriciaworby

INTRODUCTION

Every day we make 500 million new cells! That's an enormous number but it's a tiny fraction of the trillions of cells we are composed of (and the many more unicellular organisms that live in and on us). This represents an amazing opportunity of reinvention – of cellular healing and creation. 500 million chances to get the message right; from our food, our thoughts and our environment generally. We have been so inculcated with the ideas of modern medicine that health or disease is a random, genetically determined lottery (genetic determinism) that it comes as a complete paradigm shift to think of the body in this adaptive way. We need to move away from telling ourselves stories that don't support healing. This book is an attempt to show you the miracle of complexity and wonder that lie in these, the smallest component parts of your body – the cells.

We are seeing a revolution in our understanding of the body, away from a material organ-based system to a functionally and structural/informational matrix of unbelievable complexity. I chose the title 'Losing our minds'; not because this is a book about mental illness, or the diseases of ageing. It is about both of these for what joins these two seemingly disparate concepts, is the cellular matrix which links all body systems, including the brain. I chose it as it is becoming apparent to many in the healing professions that the 'mind' (i.e. the organising intelligence) is not solely (if at all) located in the brain. It exists in the gut, in the microbiome (the microbes that live in and on us) and, at a microscopic level, in the cell membrane too, where information is processed by each individual cell, communicating with its neighbours via an intelligent matrix of connective tissue called the extracellular matrix. So, 'minds' are present in each cell and loss of connectivity could be said to be loss of our inner knowing and the preclusion to all disease.

Perturbations of this dynamic system lead to disease or health depending on the adjustment made i.e. the response to the sum total of information received, sometimes called the allosatatic load. This results in a cascade of inter-related changes in hormones, peptides, neurotransmitters and a lot more besides. Virchow, the 'father of pathology' (disease) claimed 'the study of disease begins with the cell'; I would concur that health is a process not a state, largely made at the cellular level, every day. This is the basis of a health optimisation system of rebalancing as opposed to the current medical model of disease treatment via symptom suppression. It's been a long time coming, and thank goodness for an alternative, as the current system is both ineffective and bankrupt.

Chapter 1: The Cell

The Structure of the Cell

In this book I want to draw upon a *cellular* view of health and illness – a view so intricate and incredible, it defies belief. However in order to do this I have to start at the beginning of what makes living things living – the cell.

I begin by describing the basic structure of the cell to remind you how incredibly amazing and complex it is. We only began to understand these structures through the advent of new technologies, starting with the optical microscope in the 18th Century, which looked at the basic structure of a 'fixed' (essentially dead) cell though to the complex technologies of today, where it is possible to see living cells with their component parts moving, interacting and exchanging molecules. We are now able to see the 'moving parts' as it were rather than the frozen structures. See the diagram for a basic schematic of a 'typical' animal cell. Please bear in mind that there is no such thing, as all cells are highly specialized (except stem cells[i]). So, muscle cells look different to liver or heart cells for instance – the number and positioning of the various components will differ. But let's take the premise that a typical cell looks something like the one shown in the schematic overleaf.

Firstly, what is a cell? It's the basic organisational unit of a living organism – composed of proteins, lipids (fats) and carbohydrates (sugars). But these are not just assembled in a random way; they are *highly organised;* composed of structures called **organelles** suspended in a jelly-like solution called the **cytosol** or **cytoplasm** surrounded by a semi-permeable 'skin' or membrane which controls the molecules that come in and out.

---

[i] which are precursor cells and can develop into anything – hence their use in cancer treatment, muscular pain and dysfunction, etc

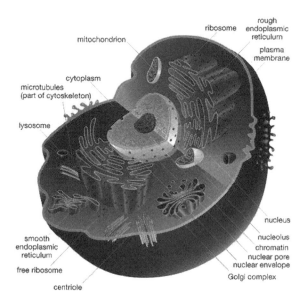

Figure 1: Schematic of a Typical Animal Cell

Within the cytosol are various structures such as the central **nucleus** containing the nuclear **DNA** (**deoxyribonucleic acid**) – the genetic information organised into coiled strings called **chromosomes**. For a long time this was considered the 'brains of the cell'. We now know it's not that simple and in fact many other structures could lay claim to that term. I am going to keep things simple for now by only describing the most important of the organelles; the first of which are **mitochondria** (energy factory, cell regulator and repository of separate DNA).

Mitochondria are at the heart of this book – as most disease is as a response to dysfunction in this organelle. Indeed they could be said to be at the heart of all disease[i]. They are one of the wonders of evolution – a symbiotic bacterium which has adapted to live permanently in the cell. I will describe them in more detail later. There is also an internal skeleton of connecting tubes called **microtubules**; these provide support and a communication highway throughout the cell as we will see later in the chapter. The rest,

---

[i]According to eminent functional medicine doctor Dr David Perlmutter

although important for the cell, are not for our discussion so, for the sake of clarity, I will omit.

Please note also this is a *diagram* (not an accurate representation) of an *animal* cell. Plant cells are somewhat different (they have energy-making structures called chloroplasts instead of mitochondria) which harness sunlight energy to transform carbon dioxide and water into carbohydrate and oxygen. This essential process is called **photosynthesis** (photo refers to the use of light for manufacture) and is a reverse of what animal cells do:

Photosynthesis

$$6CO_2 \quad +6H_2O \longrightarrow C6H_{12}O_6 \quad + \quad 6O_2$$

carbon dioxide plus water   gives carbohydrate   and oxygen

We (animals) then use these carbohydrates (sugars - usually glucose) when we eat plants to reverse that process to produce carbon dioxide when we metabolise (burn) sugars – this is called cellular **respiration** (as opposed to breathing which is a muscular process of the diaphragm and lungs – sometimes also called respiration in mammals).

Respiration

Oxygen   +   glucose —> water   +   carbon dioxide

You can see that plants and animals are mutually beneficial and linked as the *outputs* of plant processes become the *inputs* of animal ones and vice versa. We can't exist without each other.

The Cell Membrane

The cell membrane that surrounds the cell is not simply a single layered 'boundary', like a balloon skin. It is a *dynamic* junction composed of a lipid 'sandwich' between 2 protein layers. This phospholipid bi-layer is interspersed with pores and proteins which control the opening and closing of those pores, to allow the *controlled* movement of molecules in and out.

Much has been learnt about this part of the cell since it was first observed 200 or so years ago in the first microscopes. Modern imaging techniques have allowed us to observe that the cell membrane is dynamic and intelligent, not simply a passive barrier but a *gating* system. This is hugely important.

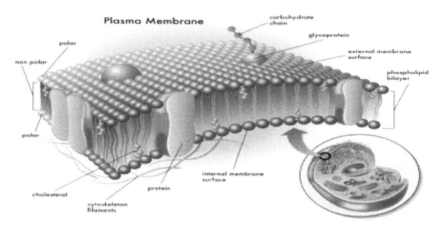

Figure 2: The Cell Membrane Lipid Bi-layer Structure

The cell biologist Bruce Lipton, in his seminal book, The Biology of Belief, talked about his 'ah-ha' moment when he discovered that the characteristics of a cell membrane mimicked exactly the characteristics of a *liquid crystal*. As I said in my second book, The World Within:

"he realised that the nature of the polar (water-loving) heads created an organic liquid crystal and the embedded proteins allowed communication of information from inside to outside. This exactly mimics the silicon chip in your computer. He believed he had found the secret of why a cell, when deprived of its nucleus (formerly considered the brains of the cell), will happily continue living until it runs out of proteins - but if the cell membrane is blocked, it dies pretty quickly. Without information flow, the cell is no longer tuned to its environment and cannot survive."

With this understanding, we see that it's not just the nuclear DNA (the blueprint) that controls the cell as we were taught, but the *information flow* from inside to outside[i], mediated by the cell membrane, that dictates cell survival (and therefore health of the organism). This is a much more *systems-based approach* than the one-way, 'top-down' model of the nucleus as the 'brains' of the cell dictating everything.

---

[i] With mitochondrial DNA input – mitos produce many metabolites which communicate the state of the organism and this is transmitted within the cell and to other cells.

Cellular Communication

Cells communicate with each other[i] to respond to their environment and send out a huge array of chemical messengers such as fragments of DNA, and other nucleotides, peptides and **cytokines**, whilst communicating with other systems such as the lymphatic and endocrine systems via hormones and neurotransmitters. Think of them as different languages but all carrying aspects of the same essential message of what's happening in the rest of the body. And then there's the energetic communication via electromagnetic signals which are poorly understood outside of physics. More on that at the end of this chapter.

How information gets from inside to outside is via structures on the outside the cell membrane called **receptors**. When a molecule 'docks' onto the receptor in a particular way, a message is sent to the inside of the cell which triggers a cascade of cellular events. How they do this is rather like putting a key into a lock (although it's much more complex). The molecule that binds to the receptor is called the **ligand** and when it binds to a receptor it triggers a host of chemical messengers inside the cell (the intracellular response). The right key fitting into the right lock only triggers this cascade which acts like a relay race to pass chemical messages on into the cell.

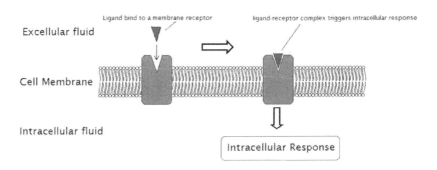

Figure 3: Cell Receptor Binding

But what happens if the messages get garbled? Then the receptors can no longer respond properly and the cell sends out more and more messages (hormones, peptides, neurotransmitters, etc) to overcome the block. This

---

[i] and with the microbes in the gut via the products of their metabolism

may deal with the problem in the short term but, after a while if the issue is not resolved, **resistance** occurs. This is where the key still fits the lock, but the lock does not turn – it's like they get stuck. This means we need more and more of the same message to produce the same effect, creating more resistance as a result. It is a downward spiral. If the messages keep misfiring then chronic illness is a logical result – the communication has turned into a cacophony or shouting match!

We see this commonly with the pancreatic hormone insulin for instance. Insulin is the hormone responsible for triggering uptake of excess blood sugars (glucose) into the cell to keep the blood sugar stable. With diets that have far more sugar in them than we need, insulin is being pumped out by the pancreas far too often and, eventually the receptors become resistant to it. Then two things happen, more insulin is pumped out as resistance develops (sometimes called **insulin resistance** or pre-diabetes) until, eventually, it stops altogether and **diabetes** results. If we can target this resistant state of pre-diabetes, diabetes itself can be prevented.

Diabetes results from a highly processed carbohydrate diet resulting in cellular dysfunction. The hormone insulin is pumped out of the pancreas when we eat sugar to divert glucose out of the blood into the liver, to lower our blood sugar (it is crucial to maintain this for health). But if it is overworked, the blood sugar dips too often and too low, driving the need to eat again to regulate symptoms (we feel shaky and irritable - often termed 'hangry'). This forces more and more insulin out of the pancreas to regulate it and we can become de-sensitised to insulin's effects, so that, just like a drug, we feel we need to consume more and more sugar. In point of fact, to improve our health we have to train ourselves to restrict sugar and carbohydrates (which acts as sugar in the body). This is easier if we find mineral and vitamin-rich foods that nourish us – then the body is less driven to feed itself with empty calories.

This is an example of the end-game of chronic disease where the body's **allostatic load** (sum total of stresses) has become too great and it can no longer adjust itself within tolerable limits to maintain **homeostasis** (a state of bodily equilibrium more correctly referred to as **allostasis** as in fact it is never stable as the prefix 'homeo' would imply but constantly being adjusted up or down in dynamic equilibrium with the environment).

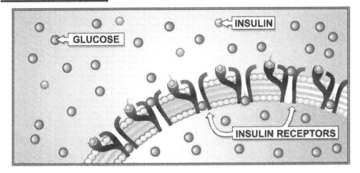

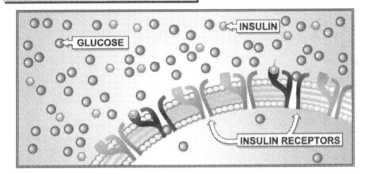

Figure 4 Insulin Resistance

Mitochondria and Insulin Resistance

Some new information about mitochondria is showing us that they are linked to insulin resistance. Remember inflammation is at the heart of all of chronic disease. **Inflammation** is a normal process of secreting inflammatory chemicals to recruit blood supply in the face of infection or damage to the organism. But chronic exposure to the messenger molecules **adipokines** (proteins produced by fat cells or adipoctyes) and cytokines are *directly toxic to mitochondria.* Unfortunately inflammation targets the insulin receptor making it less functional which drives up blood sugar which drives more inflammation – a feed forward system.

Remember mitochondria are not just power plants – as we'll see later they are directly involved in keeping a cell alive and *regulating* cell growth and inflammation via these regulatory messengers cytokines. .Mitos could be

9

considered the 'gatekeeper' for the control of inflammation or **inflammasome** as it is now called (via the mTOR pathway[i]). If the mitochondria are dysfunctional they produce more inflammatory cytokines which feedback and damage the mitos and irritate the insulin receptor which can't then lower our blood sugar, eventually causing diabetes. This has huge implications for the brain and cardiovascular system. We need to take more care of our mitos via our lifestyle: diet, exercise or stress management.

All cells have receptors for neurological or endocrine chemicals, cholinergic receptors which allow certain protein enzymes to be created and the message propagated. So, how does the message get passed to the interior of the cell to the nucleus where the genes can be turned on and off?

Protein Kinase Network - AMPK[ii]

One such cellular communication network is called the **protein kinase network**. When it is activated by cell membrane receptors, certain kinase proteins are released that carry the signal deep into the cell via a relay - each kinase handing the message to the next until they cause release of a cytokine called **NFkB**[iii]. This carries the message into the nucleus of the cell where it causes changes to the readout of the genome (sum total of genes). Here it activates the cell's gene expression to produce certain proteins with altered structure (and therefore function), creating either disease or health. It is so important that even a change in one kinase can signal a cell to go cancerous!

It is called a network for a reason: it has numerous interacting components – many routes it can follow to effect the change. This is a necessary complexity – according to Dr. Jeffrey Bland:

"the more complex a system needs to be to do its job, the greater the diversity of pathways for getting it done, the less vulnerable it will be to catastrophe. Diversity means stability."[1]

This is true of a rain forest *and* a human being. We will return to the kinase pathways again in the chapter on cancer, Chapter 8.

---

[i] The mammalian target of rapamycin (**mTOR**) pathway regulates mitochondrial oxygen consumption and oxidative capacity. The target of rapamycin (TOR) is a well conserved serine/threonine kinase network that regulates cell growth in response to nutrient status.
[ii] 5' AMP-activated protein kinase network (AMPK) to give it its full name
[iii] Transcription factor nuclear factor kappa beta

The Nucleus and Genes

The nucleus contains DNA collected into 23 string-like structures called **chromosomes** formed when the sperm of your father fused with the egg from your mother subsequently dividing to become you. It contains all their genetic information (**genes**), with one strand of DNA contributed your mother and one from your father intertwined into a structure tightly bound around proteins called **histones**. This mixing of information from mother and father gives the resultant organism 'biological variation' and is very important for survival of the species as it allows animals to adapt to environmental pressures. However, if your particular combination is not very well adapted, you will not survive to reproduce and you will die out and thus fail to spread your genes. Nature is all about survival[i].

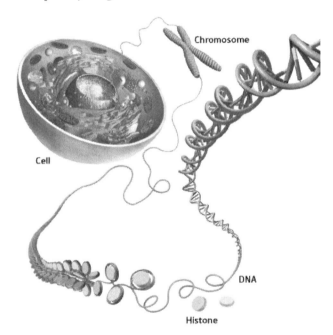

Figure 5: Chromosomes, DNA and Histone Wrapping

It used to be thought that the nucleus was the ultimate 'brains of the cell' dictating growth and every other function of the cell. However, a strange

---

[i]Though not, as Darwin put it, survival of the fittest i.e. competitive. It is more like survival of the most cooperative i.e. collaborative. The more adaptive the organism to its environment the more likely it is to survive.

observation by cell biologists that 'de-nucleated' cells could function very well without a nucleus puzzled them and challenged that view. We will now look at some other contenders for that role.

Mitochondria: Functions and Structure

Mitochondria are tiny organelles (intracellular structures) that exist in almost every cell of the body (except red blood cells). They are sometimes called the 'powerhouse' of the cell, as they produce energy, but in fact they are far more than that as I will discuss later.

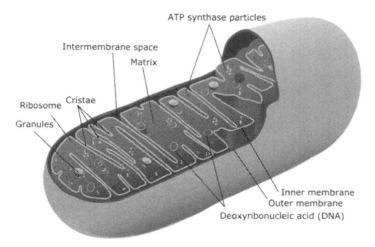

Figure 6: Mitochondrial Structure

Energy production

Energy production is essential for every process that happens in the body and mitochondria are the organelles that do it. Each cell has between 100 and 100,000 mitochondria (except red blood cells which carry oxygen around the body)[i]. Each mitochondrion consists of a lozenge shape structure surrounded by an external membrane (like the cell itself) and many convoluted internal membranes which increase the surface area for reactions to take place. And, of course given our earlier discussion on the importance of the membrane to cellular intelligence, you will perhaps not be surprised to know that these membranes have other functions besides

---

[i] Red blood cells dont' have any mitos as oxygen would be too damaging to their function. Interestingly they have no nucleus either presumably for the same reason.

energy production. But let's deal with that first as it is important to cellular functioning.

The molecular unit of energy is **adenosine triphosphate (ATP)**, a highly structured molecule with many double bonds between atoms (which makes it a good holder of information[i]) and 3 phosphate groups attached (which are water-soluble which is important for how chemical reactivity – sometimes called the 'polar' head).

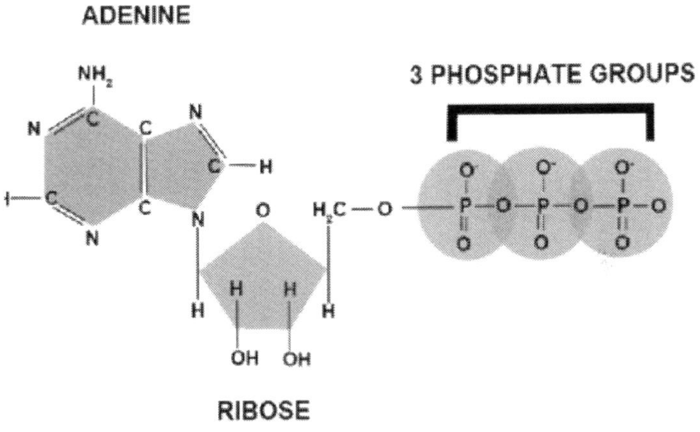

Figure 7: An ATP Molecule

ATP is produced by a complex exchange of electrons (negatively charged subatomic particles shown as e-in chemical convention), protons (positively charged H^+) and photons (elementary light particles – not shown in the diagram[ii]). These subatomic particles pass through a complex of membrane-embedded proteins called the **electron transport chain (ETC)**. This incredible complex structure is beautifully co-ordinated to produce the energy we need from oxygen. It has often been likened to a factory production line which is a useful (though limited) analogy.

---

[i]Double bonds in a ring structure are resonant- electrons are held more tightly and they vibrate in a resonant way – they are much like a liquid crystal.
[ii]Energy production is a *quantum process* not a mechanistic one as this diagram suggests so we must view the wave function of light as being important in this process.

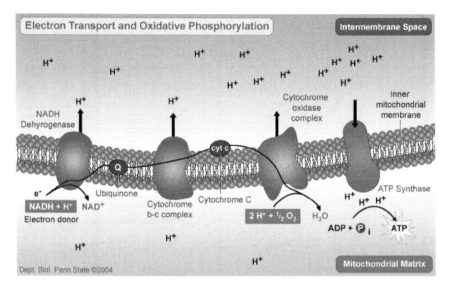

Figure 8: The Electron Transport Chain

Note that we have the same bi-layer (sandwich) membrane structure as the external cell membrane (Figure 3) but the ETC lies on the convoluted inner membranes *within the mitochondrion* (see Figure 6 to remind yourself where these are). Mitos have a looped inner membrane structure to maximise the surface area for reaction. In this diagram above, we have focused *on one section* of the inner membrane to simplify it.

If you remember ever doing experiments in school with how water always leaches out from the most concentrated solution to the least concentrated (osmosis), so is true of protons and electrons. This so-called 'concentration gradient' helps to drive the 'engine' of the ETC and it's an incredibly efficient process called **oxidative phosphorylation.** This was bequeathed to us by the bacteria that first fused with our primitive cells to become our mitochondria[i]. Without those early bacteria we would never have come to be as sophisticated as we are - our energy systems were simply not productive enough to drive our complexity. Moreover, we have just begun to realise that light helps drive the process too by a means so mysterious it is only now becoming elucidated but which we now know to be quantum in nature. It is a truly wondrous thing to behold..

---

[i] Mitochondria are remnants of bacteria that fused with us hundreds of thousands of years ago now living as permanent symbiotic (mutually beneficial) residents!

However there is a problem the organism has to solve. As part of our energy production process, dangerous **free radicals** (or sometimes also called **reactive oxygen species** or **ROS–** think of them as 'rust') are produced, an excess of which causes cellular damage. This is why we need a good supply of **antioxidant** molecules (especially those from plants – and the fat-soluble vitamins A, D, E and K) to help *dampen* the ROS production, like oil does with rust. There are problems if these ROS are allowed to run rampant without this so-called 'quenching' by antioxidants; co-ordination of ROS and anti-oxidants is very important to prevent premature ageing. However, it is the *balance* not the overall numbers that are important. You can have too many antioxidants too as we have discovered with over-dosing certain fat-soluble vitamins[i].

Mitochondrial Intra-cellular Communication

According to the latest thinking, mitochondria are not just mechanical powerhouses, blindly producing energy like a factory production line, but complex structures which influence vital bodily functions such as memory and ageing, through to combating stress and disease[2]. It has been said that:

"mitochondria control many more cellular functions.. such as cell death (apoptosis), cell proliferation (growth), autophagy (self-destruction), cell differentiation (making different types of cell) and aging. Perhaps the mitochondrial network is actually the 'brains' of the cell, controlling much of the cell's processes, including activities of the nucleus."[26]

So this is another claim to be the brains of the cell besides the nucleus and the cell membrane! Mitochondria are present in every cell except red blood cells and are essential for life as they produce the energy that every process needs. They are particularly needed in nerve conduction, being present at the ends of nerve fibres in large numbers in order to facilitate the release of neurotransmitters and the electrochemical signal along the nerve fibre (axon). We return to this in the chapter on neuro-degeneration (Chapter 7).

Mitochondria are certainly very interesting structures from a genetic point of view; they have their own DNA or '**genome**' inherited from the maternal line (your mother, her mother, etc) only. Unlike the chromosome (**nuclear DNA** – a double helix), the mitochondrial genome is a small

---

[i] In a famous study of people with lung cancer, excess dosing with artificial vitamin A actually made outcomes worse. However this is complicated by the type of vitamin A, the dosing schedules and excess amounts which are not what the body recognises.

circular DNA molecule with multiple copies of **mitochondrial DNA (mtDNA)** in the **matrix** (liquid middle) of each mitochondrion.

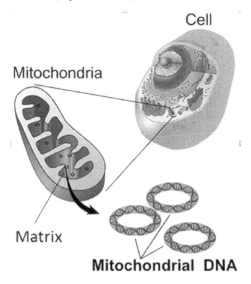

Figure 9: Mitochondrial DNA

This mtDNA can talk to the nuclear DNA (chromosomes)in that cell and *both* can communicate to the DNA in other cells and **microbial DNA (mDNA)** in the gut and other places (**microbiome).** This **'cross-talk'** is really important in terms of body function, health and wellbeing.

Consider then, that the messages your mother received during her lifetime are likely transmitted **epigenetically[i]** to you (and so on down the generations) by your mtDNA. Unlike nuclear DNA, there is no mixing of mother and father's genes, so it has a very different and specific message. If your mother was stressed by her upbringing or circumstances, then likely that changes the expression of her DNA and this gets inherited by you. Stress can be *epigenetically inherited* therefore. An amazing thought!

It is the interaction of all the different signalling molecules: peptides, ATP, cytokines, mitochondrial, nuclear and microbial DNA[ii] that gives the cell the sum total of information. It is a communication system of immense

[i]Epigenetics is the interaction of genes and environment; stress can be transmitted this way for many generations.
[ii]The true definition of the microbiome, a term which truly describes the *genetic component* of your microbial partners, which is *at least* 100x your own!

16

complexity which responds to minute signals from its environment on an ongoing basis. It is thus minutely susceptible to the quality of that environment. As I have said in my book The World Within:

"This communication system gets fouled by toxicity both within and outside the cells. For example, with an inflamed cell membrane, hormones can't dock onto receptors and can't deliver the message into the cell or get into the cell itself. Cells become inflamed and toxic causing inflammatory cytokines to be released. At this lower level of inflammation, the membranes of the mitochondrion become inflamed and the cell can't make energy - ATP production is affected. If that goes on long enough, the immune system which has priority for your energy, gets mixed up and can't identify friend from foe and auto-immune disease results.[3]"

So disease, particularly auto-immune disease, is a direct result of cellular toxicity. This is a really important understanding which few in the medical profession understand. Auto-immune disease is simply described as a random unfortunate event, where the immune system goes AWOL for no apparent reason[i]. This doesn't make sense. The systems-based view of the body, which I am putting together here, would see this as a *failure of coordination*, which can be understood as a logical result of blockages in the system, not a random event. The body is never random, it is intelligent and what's more – it is a quantum biological system. Let me explain what I mean by that statement.

Firstly you should understand that there has long been a battle going on in science between a matter-driven, mechanistic view of the body, and an energetic, complex view which sees the body as part of a larger system including the earth itself. This latter view is gaining ground but there is still a large body of established opinion against it, not least because if people were shown they can harness this energy themselves, they may have no need for pharmaceutical (matter-driven) medicine.

ATP: an Intra-cellular Antenna

The simplified biomolecular (matter-driven) view of the mitochondrial energy molecule would have it that it is a molecular 'pawn' to be passed around various parts of the cell being recycled, releasing energy as it does

---

[i] When I was diagnosed with Hashimoto's thyroiditis my GP said to me in answer to my question why me maybe 'it's just one of those things'! No it's not.

so. But there is an emerging theory that ATP is more than an energy molecule. According to Dr Heinrich Kremer and his Cell Synthesis Theory:

> "ATP serves as an 'antennae molecule' for the reception and relaying of resonance information from the morphogenetic background field[i] ." Foods are part of that source of information; how they are grown, what colour they are and their rich and diverse interaction with the soil and sunlight. It is a huge shock to realise that the information is not derived just from molecules i.e. matter-driven. This is because light is not a particle but a wave of potentiality (though it can behave as a particle or 'photon' when observed)."

Thus ATP and many biological molecules of respiration and photosynthesis are not cogs in a material machine, but quantum transfer intermediaries. It's a new **quantum biology** understanding which is gaining ground, as quantum physics begins to invade biology.

Cell Structure - Microtubule Network

The cell is not simply a bag of jelly; it is highly structured. The cell 'jelly' or cytosol isn't just liquid but a complex matrix of little microscopic tubules which helps support the cell (a bit like the skeleton does the body) and help to transmit information and molecules around it. Here is a micrograph (microscopic photograph) of the microtubule network (stained with fluorescent dye) in an animal cell.

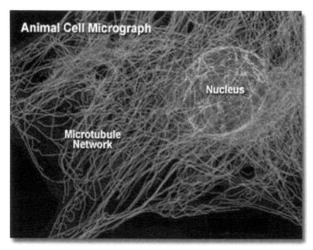

Figure 10: Microtubule Network of the Cell

---

[i] This is the vibrational field which is now understood to be everywhere and out of which matter emerges.

This network has an important value in sensing and protecting the cell as well as a special function when it is time for the cell to divide.

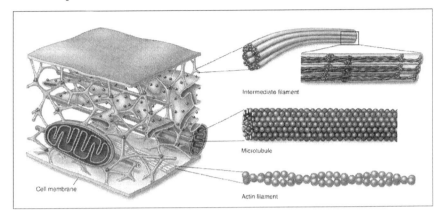

Figure 11: Microtubule Structure

Cell Growth and Division

In order to grow, an organism's cells must split and divide into so-called 'daughter' cells. The reason is that the cells eventually grow so large they don't have enough surface area (on the membrane) to support themselves – there is a balance here between size and efficiency. The larger the central cytoplasmic core, the more surface area is needed to support it nutritionally and, as the cell grows, the surface area reduces in proportion to the volume (think about this and you'll see it's true). So, at a certain crucial point its surface area is not large enough to support the movement of crucial food in and wastes out and the cell stops growing and prepares instead to divide.

This is not a simple splitting like you would imagine cutting something into two (except in single celled organisms!) In most multi-cellular organisms (that's us) it's a highly co-ordinated process – necessarily so because of the complexity of the structures in the cell. The first problem is how to split the genetic material in the chromosomes as they are located in the nucleus as we've seen. They are protected from the oxidation in the cell by the **nuclear membrane** (another membrane that surrounds the nucleus).

During cell division (a process called **mitosis**) they have to be exposed in order to be replicated by the dissolution of the nuclear membrane, pulled apart into 2 halves to opposite ends of the cell as it divides. Eventually the nucleus will reform in the two daughter cells each with half the divided chromosomes as a new complement of genes.

The microtubules are intimately involved in this process as they form the lattice along which the chromosomes are pulled. They guide the chromosomes and form the mechanism by which they are divided without damage. It is a complex process which I can't cover in detail here but as a quick summary study the diagram below.

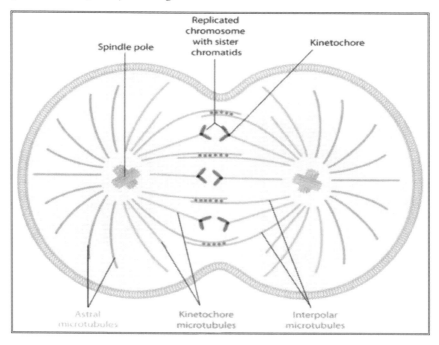

Figure 12: Mitosis with Microtubules

As with all diagrams, this makes it look much less magnificent than it really is. Hence I include a slide of stained cells to show the various stages of actual dividing cells. Note the gradual separation of the two halves of the chromosomes to opposite poles of the cell before division. It really is magnificent!

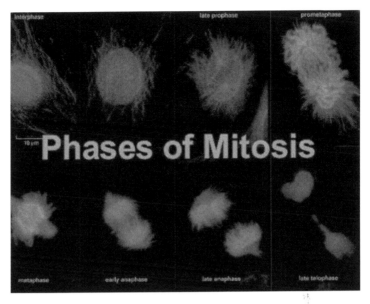

Figure 13: Phases of Mitosis

Tubulin proteins which make up microtubules are polar molecules[i] with a particular quality of being able to form geometric lattices which quantum biologists Roger Penrose and Stuart Hameroff have postulated "may support energy transfer, which could be important for biological signalling and communication essential to living processes."[73]

We know from the work done on the artificial carbon compound graphene, that when ordered structures such as lattices are layered in a particular way, then extraordinary features such as superconductivity start to appear[4]. Could not the structures of the cell also perform this quantum 'electron tunneling' effect? The jury is still out on this but it's an intriguing thought which leads us nicely on to other quantum effects within the cell.

Quantum Cellular Effects

Some cellular properties that are perhaps less well understood even by cell scientists – steeped as they are in the traditional **biomolecular model** which ignores energy as information. According to Harry Massey, founder of innovative company NES Health:

---

[i] They have both positive and negatively charged ends which makes them align in particular ways. Water, tubulin and phosphate are examples of polar molecules.

"A lot of the phenomena in our body cannot be explained with biochemistry alone... they cannot happen that quickly. e.g. coordinating when we're running cannot be accounted for by the traditional model of biochemistry. Not only that, but the energy that our body produces cannot be explained from the amount of energy the mitochondria produce. The mitochondria only produce a small fraction of our body's energy and the rest is explained with **bioenergetics**. Cells do have biochemical receptors but they also have receptors for energy waves or, if you like, the energy field. It's through those cell receptors that the body is able to react so quickly. ..There are trillions of reactions happening every single second in your body which biochemistry basically can't orchestrate. However, an energy field and the information and the instructions that are carried in the energy field *can* orchestrate that instantaneously."[i]

These are what we know so far of how the cell functions at a quantum level i.e. very small (smaller than atoms), non-linear, 'spooky' reactions that seem to eschew space and time limitations. You may have heard of quantum physics as a way of describing the world of very small or large things like the particles formed in the Hadron Collider and black holes in space. For a long while, the quantum world wasn't thought to operate in living systems – it was believed it was too wet and warm. We now know this isn't true. One of the first discoveries that hinted at this and solved one of the mysteries of biology was that water operates differently in living systems.

The Fourth Phase of Water

This is another recent discovery which is driving our new understanding of cellular processes: the nature of biological water. You've no doubt learned that water has 3 phases: gas, liquid or solid but we now know there is a fourth phase called the *gel phase*, which forms exclusively in biological structures. This water possesses an extraordinary property of forming an **Exclusion Zone** *(EZ)*: a negatively charged interior layer surrounded by protons. This EZ (gel-state) water contains lipophilic (fat loving) tubules create a highly negative hydration gradient by ejecting protons (positively-charged particles). It seems to be an informational structure which can flip between different quantum states which has been hypothesised as a mechanism for quantum processes which would otherwise require too much energy to happen.

---

[i] Harry talks about bioenergetics on the NES website. The programme and training are very comprehensive but expensive

Suffice to say water is a quantum informational molecule[i] essential to life and the incorporation into tissues changes its properties. This layer acts like a battery and, with infra-red energy (from metabolic processes and light), helps to propel biological processes like blood flow. It may even *hold memory* as an inevitable effect of a quantum system i.e. polarised, entangled (interconnected) system which holds information. This is true, also, of DNA, Vitamin D, and all the **chromophores** (double bond rich, light harvesting molecules) present in the body.

Living systems have adapted to optimise quantum effects by the use of the properties of this fourth phase of water[ii]. Gerald Pollock is the researcher who investigated this property and has been largely responsible for the dissemination and application of this theory. More is yet to be discovered in this field of quantum biology, a truly interdisciplinary field which unites physics, chemistry, microbiology and medicine. It is mind-boggling to think that something as simple as water could operate so intelligently under biological conditions.

Our Electromagnetic Nature and Other Mysteries

We know that we are electrical beings as well as material ones and that energy doesn't only come from food - since energy is linked to electron transfer in the body, it can also come from the earth via grounding. When we used to walk barefoot or in leather soles, we were naturally connected with the earth. Now that we travel and work in metal /glass boxes, with electrically charged computers and lights, and walk with insulated (plastic) shoes /sneakers, we no longer receive electron transfer with the earth. This grounding (earthing) has profound implications. The earth is negatively charged and we humans tend to be positively charged with free radicals and heavy metals from pollution, so contact with the earth is really important.

According to the work of respected cardiologist Stephen Sinatra[iii], when you walk barefoot you take in millions of electrons and this quenches the dangerous free radicals or ROS (remember – 'rust'). There is a lot of

---

[i] Quantum theory dictates some very strange qualities: action at a distance – a change in one sub-atomic particle like an electron causes a response in a linked but distance particle, superposition – a particle can be both matter or energy but never both at the same time. If you find its position then it becomes matter but when you aren't looking it can be just a probability of existing, not a material thing. Very odd stuff

[ii] I refer you to the book by Jim Al-Khaleli 'Life on the Edge for a fuller discussion

[iii] See https://heartmdinstitute.com for more info

information about this in the medical literature[i] such that it has been called 'electric nutrition'[5], so it is important to understand and incorporate into your life. It seems this shifts the **autonomic nervous system** via vagal stimulation and improves heart rate variability (a functional measure of autonomic health) which I covered in chapter 2.

So, I hope I have hinted at the sheer magnificence of the cell – there is much I can't cover here. I'll leave you with the words of Dr Jon Lieff:

"The eukaryote cell is, in fact, an enormous civilization with many buildings, rooms, pathways, transport systems, free living symbiotic bacteria called mitochondria travelling to where energy is needed, and elaborate machinery of many types with thousands of interlocking proteins. The nucleus is highly guarded at the entrance pores and the DNA is protected by elaborate large molecules that wind the DNA around spools and then cover it, making it very hard for invaders to find. Despite all of this, microbes find the DNA and manipulate it for their own purposes. The cell is constantly being assaulted by invaders, and most are eliminated by specific mechanisms the cell has evolved for each different type of virus and bacteria. How can we not say that this enormously complex eukaryote cell defending against countless different microbes and strategies does not exhibit great intelligence?"

I'll leave you to ponder.. In the next Chapter we will look at the systems that maintain this intelligence.

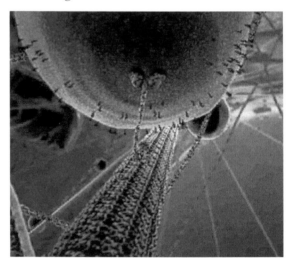

Figure 14: A Quantum Cellular Network

---

[i] Over 1700 articles in Pub Med currently

Chapter 2: The Body as a System

Having looked at the smallest identifiable living system - the cell, (omitting viruses and bacteria as we are concentrating on human structures), we now turn to the 'bigger picture'. We have been taught that the body is a series of independent structures which exist in isolation; modern medicine is predicated on this notion with its idea of medical 'specialties'. Doctors train in general medicine and then they specialise in areas such as rheumatology (joints), endocrinology (hormones), etc. The problem with this approach is that they become so focused on learning one area in detail that they lose sight of the interconnections. The body is not constructed in this way – each part is linked to every other part, and the cross-talk between systems is such that you cannot make a change in one system without affecting the other. This is the nature of **systems biology** – a new field that is informing a new, more biologically accurate medical approach called **systems** or **functional medicine**[i].

In this approach we see any illness as *an imbalance of the system* – the whole is the sum of the parts and cannot be divorced from them. As the eminent mitochondrial researcher Robert Naviaux has said: "every chronic disease is actually a whole body disease – a systems problem – that cannot be solved using this (old functionally separate) paradigm". In this new understanding, in order to effect healing we have to go to the *root cause* and re-balance the weakest part of the system so all the others can automatically rebalance themselves. This is a radical departure from current medical practice[ii] and one that increasing numbers of patients are turning to as the old method becomes less and less effective[iii].

---

[i]Herbert Schimmel the German physiologist, first coined this term which may surprise you!
[ii]Although it's fair to say that Ancient Chinese Medicine knew this very well and so did conventional medicine of the 1920's and 30's – albeit piecemeal.
[iii] According to Zach Bush, MD, in 1960 4% of the US population had a chronic disease,

The body system is incredibly complex and highly organized. Remember, the more *complex* a system is the more options it has in fighting threats to the system. This is the basis of **complexity theory** and sees the body as a collection of systems which interface.

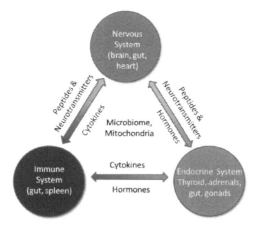

Figure 15: Immune, Nervous and Endocrine System Interface

In order to fully understand this approach we need to introduce some of these interconnections which I now describe.

The Extracellular Matrix (ECM)

We are making large strides in our understanding of how a live human body works as opposed to studying cadavers (thanks to the new live scanning technologies available to us). However, there is one element that has eluded us til now - the matrix that links all the cells of the body together in a structured, informational way. This **extracellular matrix (ECM)**, as it is called, is a "complex meshwork of cross-linked proteins providing both biophysical and biochemical cues that are important regulators of cell proliferation, survival, differentiation and migration"[6].

now 43% of children have one! Something is very wrong...

26

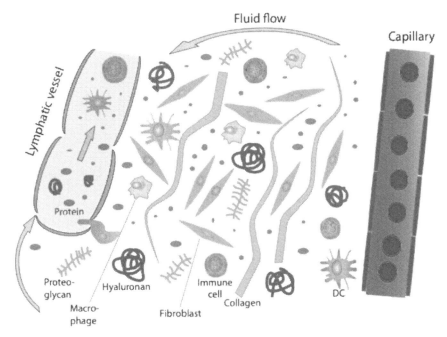

Figure 16: The Extracellular Matrix

ECM Structure and function

It consists of connective tissue (collagen fibres), lymphatic and blood vessels and various immune cells integral to the function and behavior of cells. In particular it controls the life cycle of the cell, how growth factors are utilised, and therefore whether the tissues develop pathology (disease) or not. It is composed of a mixture of specialised immune cells called mast cells, structural components called fibroblasts suspended in a watery liquid containing glyco-protein molecules called **glycoaminoglycans** (**GAGs.**) These are protein-based sugars containing **glycine**, a vital amino acid for the body and one particularly associated with connective tissue. GAGs seem to act as transmitter molecules which allow information to be transmitted throughout the ECM which signals health or disease. These GAG molecules are vital to how the ECM operates.

Glycine, the other component of the GAG, has another important function; it is one of the amino acids that is used in the synthesis of **glutathione,** which is our most powerful intracellular antioxidant

27

(detoxification) system. Without enough glutathione we cannot neutralise some of the inflammatory molecules produced by natural energy production in the mitochondria as I've already described. The tissues are flooded with degraded molecules which cannot be repaired. The informational matrix becomes dysfunctional; the information is disorganised and disrupted.

This understanding of how cells are bathed in and organized by the ECM has been known about since its discovery in the 1950's by the German physiologist Alfred Pissinger. His investigations demonstrated that we couldn't consider the cells in isolation, as cellular biologists had been doing.[i] He and other (mostly German) scientists developed the concepts of the holistic functioning of the cell matrix which has been recently characterized as the **matrisome.** This is current terminology for the characteristic components of the network in different disease states – a sort of biological inventory. This inventory of metabolic output is being recognised as the mediator of both bioenergetics and functional medicine understanding. It is integral to function and behavior of the cell e.g. .life cycle, and growth.

When there are problems with the ECM, certain disorders arise. According to researcher Michael McEvoy, it is a "meeting place and battle ground and communicative epicenter where neuro-endocrine and immune systems meet to create a homeostatic balance".

Where there is degradation to the matrix the connective tissues cannot function. Hence we are seeing a rise in connective tissue disorders like arthritis**, scleroderma, Depuytrens contracture** (a degradation of the tissue by specialist **metalloproteinase enzymes (MMP**s) which we cover again later. But, even more importantly, we are finding that the immune cells within the ECM are no longer able to communicate properly with the rest of the body they become hyper-reactive and this leads to auto-immune diseases of a much more serious, systemic nature (e.g. RA, lupus, etc). It is involved in all responses to toxicity (including mould), and particularly **chronic inflammatory response syndrome (CIRS**– formerly called histamine intolerance), due to activation of a destructive enzyme called metalloproteinases (MMP-9), which bores a hole in the ECM beginning the degradation of the collagen fibres allowing more immune cells to infiltrate.

---

[i] and continue to do.. science is often based on a reductionist, isolated study of cells in petri dishes rather than in living systems as these are more difficult to study.

Symptoms of peripheral neuropathy are: tissue hypoxia (discolouration of finger tips, etc). Various growth factors (IGF, VEGF, etc) have binding and maturation sites in the glycoproteins, so if these are being degraded they can't mature and we see symptoms including loss of cognitive function interestingly.

RCCX gene complex

Some people have a genetic higher predisposition to these issues e.g. if they have joint hypermobility their ability to synthesise collagen has been impaired. This results in certain characteristic diseases e.g. **Ehlers-Danlos Syndrome (EDS)** and **Marfan syndrome**. These are all highly linked to a gene complex on Chromosome 6 called the **RCCX gene complex**. This exciting new discovery links sensitivity to cortisol (and therefore stress) and chronic inflammation by the deficient gene products (or adaptive depending on your viewpoint)[i]. The mutations in this gene cluster cause a deficiency of certain proteins resulting in tissue hypoxia, weak muscle tone, POTS, mast cell activation syndrome (related to histamine intolerance)/CFS/ME, problems with blood clotting, PCOS etc. Mast cells (a form of immune cell) may then accumulate, breaking down the structure of the ECM which normally requires fibroblasts to spin out the 'web' of the matrix components to keep everything stable. Environmental toxins play a big role - GAGs are negatively charged so attract positive metals like aluminium and cadmium, which bond to the sulphate tails of GAG's (as does glyphosate as we'll see later).

How can we support basic matrix function? Marine red algae has been shown in some research to inhibit MMP-9 and to increase collagen synthesis; some individuals with joint hyper-mobility taking sulphated polysaccharides from marine red algae and increased vitamin C showed 30% less hyper-mobility in finger joints after 10 – 14 days. And in addition inflammatory markers like C-reactive protein (CRP) are completely normalised too! Gentle exercise and body work also help to normalize function. We will return to this in Chapter 3 when we look at toxicity and the **Cell Danger Response**.

---

[i]For more information on this see rccxandillness.com ?. It explains the underlying pathophysiology of chronic fatiguing illnesses with so many overlapping features (EDS-HT, CFS, Chronic Lyme Disease, Fibromyalgia, toxic mold, Epstein Barr Infection, POTS, etc.).

Fascia

Fascia and the ECM are often used synonymously but are *not* the same thing. Fascia includes the higher connective tissues structure of the body (containing ECM). Fascia has largely been ignored until very recently as playing any role at all in the body. It used to be routinely removed from cadavers when investigating anatomy but it turns out it is the connective tissue that gives us our integrity. Without fascia the muscles and bones would collapse into a heap. Fascia is wrapped around every bone, muscle, nerve fibre and blood vessel. It includes all the collagenous-based soft-tissues in the body, including the cells that create and maintain that network of the extra-cellular matrix (ECM). This is set within structural materials, a **colloid**[i] suspension of the proteins **elastin** and **collagen** set within the ECM or ground substance (containing the polymer **hyaluronic acid** that make it more like a liquid crystal matrix which can respond to changes in temperature and strain by extending or contracting and changing its structure from a liquid to a solid. It also possesses an ability to transmit electrical current when stimulated – called the **piezo-electric effect**. Thus it is actually a 'cell signalling' matrix that co-ordinates disparate body structures "creating networks within networks"[7] and may be implicated in cancer too as we will discuss in Chapter 8.

Because fascia provides the basic substrate through which nerve interactions happen, it responds to stress and tension. So when stimulated by the autonomic nervous system (ANS) through sympathetic and parasympathetic innervations, it responds to body messages of challenge or support. When we are feeling overwhelmed and stressed, our fascia tightens and the message of constriction it sends to the matrix is one of slow down and threat. Additionally, after an injury, it's common for fascia to constrict around the injury in order to provide structured protection, tightening the whole fascial system and potentially causing pain and discomfort in an area of the body not associated with the injury[ii].

The gut has its own enteric (gut) nervous system intertwined with the fascia[iii]. A part of the autonomic nervous system (ANS), it functions without us

---

[i] A colloid is a very interesting state which can act as both liquid and solid under different conditions. When poked with a sharp instrument you can pierce it like a liquid but when you put a flat weight on it, it acts as a solid being able to support the weight without dispersal.
[ii] This is known as 'referred pain' and happens in predictable pathways known as trigger point patterns.

thinking about it, but requires communication between the structural mechano-system of the fascia and the ANS sympathetic and parasympathetic nerve fibres that run through it. There is a two way communication between these two systems. Generally, sympathetic stimulation ('fight and flight' - our stress response), inhibits gastrointestinal secretions and causes the digestive tract to constrict or close down. Parasympathetic stimuli (our 'rest and digest' system) stimulates digestive activities – hence we need a balance of the two for good gut motility and digestion. Being relaxed and in gratitude when we eat helps our digestion.

The Interstitium and Acupuncture

The **interstitium** is the space which holds the ECM, and its relevance has only very recently been explored. There is a great deal of excitement as it seems to operate as an organ system even though it is located throughout the body. The Chinese had a concept in their ancient medicine system (TCM) that is called the 'triple burner' which they regarded as 'the organ that includes everything but has no form'. According to innovative British acupuncturist Dr. Daniel Keown, the interstitium could be the modern physiological equivalent. It often holds heavy metals particularly aluminium and glyphosate in its tissues and is thus very vulnerable to infection from diseases such as the bacteria of Lyme Disease (which are attracted to the metals). It is very exciting to explore the remarkable relationship between these ancient systems and a more modern understanding of the body.

If you look at the body tissue through an embryological lens i.e. how the body develops *in utero*, you can trace the development of the tissues (particularly fascia and the ECM) along lines which correspond to the 'meridian lines' of Chinese Medicine. US researcher Alfred Pissinger's explored the use of acupuncture and the effect that it has on matrix function. He was able to demonstrate clearly how the insertion of a single acupuncture needle into connective tissue caused what he calls **leukocytolysis** or the breakdown of billions of white blood cells. Instantaneously they begin to degrade, releasing all kinds of chemicals and essentially creating a 'broadband communication network' from the site of

---

[iii]Embryologically, the gut and the brain form from the same tissues which then migrate to opposite poles of the developing embryo. They share many characteristics including a single layer of cells which separate it from the blood supply (gut lining and the blood brain barrier respectively).

injection to the distant parts of the matrix[i]. This could be one of the ways in which information is transmitted throughout the body.

So when we understand that the ECM is an *informational system*, we can use this understanding to find out what goes wrong to cause disease. Let's see how it intersects with the other systems of the body to process information.

Nutrients and the fascia

CBD Oil

Cannabidiol (CBD) oil is the non-psychoactive component of the hemp plant, recently becoming very popular in relieving pain, depression and anxiety. It seems to do this by regulating the HPA axis (stress response) as well as promoting **GABA-inergic signalling**[ii] to turn off the sympathetic fight or flight response. However, CBD has proved particularly useful to those that have this particular phenotype of matrix dysregulation. It seems to act in similar ways to **low dose naltrexone (LDN)**, which many in health-conscious circles have been using with some degree of benefit. It seems to modulate the pain response via altering pain receptors[8]. Its application in emotional memory and learned fear (phobias) are also impressive[9].

Vitamin C

Vitamin C (ascorbate) is integral in the function of the ECM. Ascorbate plays an important role as an antioxidant in the endothelium especially. And so when you have **scurvy** (acute lack of vitamin C) for example, that is basically as a result of collagen break-down. We also need copper. Copper and vitamin C are integral to the processes of collagen synthesis. There's a form of hyper-mobility called **Ehlers-Danlos Syndrome (EDS)** that is linked to a deficiency of lysyl oxidase- a transport protein for copper in the connective tissue. Observations of people with hyper-mobility, show indications of low copper, either low serum or plasma copper, or low **VEGF (vascular endothelial growth factor)**. If they then take

---

[i] When I've had acupuncture by a trained Traditional Chinese medicine practitioner, I can feel this electrical 'flow' around my body. Not so when needles are placed just anywhere.
[ii] GABA or Gamma amino butyric acid is the relaxation neurotransmitter which is needed to balance the stress response

supplemental copper in higher amounts under supervision it can actually have a benefit to the regulation of some of these functions.

The Immune and Lymphatic Systems

These are perhaps the most misunderstood systems of the human body – and so vital to our health.

Lymphatic system

No nutrition gets to the cell without the lymphatic system. It's the transport system as well as a battleground for the immune system. It is composed of a network of nodes (storage areas), and vessels which transport the lymph fluid around the body. Unlike the cardiovascular (blood) system, it doesn't have a heart to pump fluid around and relies on movement of the body as well as a pacemaker system in the larger collecting vessels[10]. It is far from a passive system though, as it is innervated by the autonomic nervous system and responds to many signals from the body, both nervous and chemical. One of the main functions of lymphatic vessels is to return fluid which has been extruded from cells, distributing proteins, cholesterol and cells themselves back into the blood circulation, particularly in un-muscled areas of the body. A blocked lymphatic system is implicated in both cardiovascular disease and cancer for that reason.

As with all the systems I have been describing, it does not exist in isolation; it is in constant communication with the immune system. Indeed, the maturation of our **dendritic cells** (part of the immune system in the gut which present **antigens** to our T-cells) is largely dependent upon what's going on in the lymphatic fluids which run through the connective tissue. The gut lining is only one cell thick and lymphatic vessels run just under the surface so they are intimately connected.

Immune System

The immune system is incredibly complex and is best thought of as various 'forces' like the army, navy, special forces, etc which protect our body from attack in a highly co-ordinated way. Now bear with me, I am going to try to make this simple. If you do nothing else read the diagrams.

33

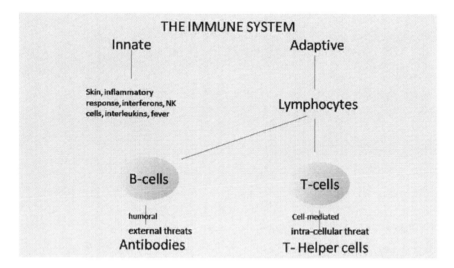

Figure 17: The Different Arms of the Immune System

Innate Immune System

The immune system consists of 2 basic arms; the **innate** system which is the first line *non-specific* but a fast-response defence system which comes online within minutes of encountering a microbial threat. It consists of physical and chemical barriers which are present at birth. It includes:

"the epithelial and mucosal linings of our respiratory and GI tracts, as well as our skin. These act as physical and chemical barriers against pathogens. Cells known as **macrophages** also play a large role in innate immunity. Macrophages recognize bacterial or viral components such as **lipopolysaccharide (LPS)** or double-stranded RNA (dsRNA), via special receptors known as **Toll-like receptors (TLRs)**. TLR activation cause macrophages to secrete cytokines (cell signalling molecules), as well as to phagocytose (gobble up) the infected cells."[11]

Adaptive Immune Response

The slower **adaptive** immune system is then activated, which deals with microbial and non-microbial threats that have to be encountered to be learnt. It consists of the more classically understood organs of the lymph nodes, spleen, and mucosal associated lymphoid tissue. This system is the most complex as you'd imagine as it has to remember certain properties of the **antigen** in order to make sure should it encounter it again it will react more quickly. Thus it is said to have memory!

Initially it is primed by the mother's microbiome and then by what it encounters in early life. That's why childhood infections like measles and mumps, etc are quite important to help the child's immune system to recognise such pathogens so it can identify and kill them in future (the child becomes **immunised**). Proponents of vaccines use this fact when including live or dead bacterial or viral particles to artificially stimulate the immune reaction. The problem can be that individual children react differently to these artificial mixtures of biologic and chemical vaccines (some contain **adjuvants** like aluminium, or mercury to provoke the immune system further). And the immune system may react differently to these artificial concoctions compared to how it would to native pathogens. Hence immunization and vaccination are not the same thing although often referred to synonymously.

Adaptive immunity has various lymphocytes (white blood cells) to do the job which are again divided into two arms:

1. **Humoral** system (**B-cells**) –deals with external threats via specific proteins called **antibodies**.
2. **Cell-mediated** (**T cells**) – deals with intra-cellular invasion or dysfunction (e.g. as in cancer or viruses).

This more cell-mediated immune system has a variety of different types of T-cells formed in a gland called the **Thymus** (hence 'Th'). It is the interplay of these cell types that orchestrate the adaptive immune response. There are various **Th cell** types that form from a Th0 cell (undifferentiated **stem cell**) depending on what threat is present and what cytokines are produced (each type has a characteristic cytokine profile).

1. Th1 cells tend to generate responses against intracellular parasites such as bacteria and viruses,
2. Th2 cells produce immune responses against helminthes (worms) and other extracellular parasites
3. Th17cells tend to be against extracellular bacteria and fungi as well as involved in auto-immunity.
4. Finally T-regulatory cells (T-Regs) are, as you would expect, to do with maintaining balance and regulation of the immune response.

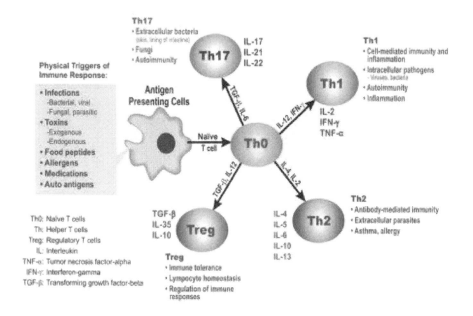

Figure 18: The Adaptive Immune System

Cellular immunity

Having defined the immune system as traditionally understood I now want to introduce you to a new concept that is only just becoming known. Each cell has a contribution to make to immunity – we call it **cellular immunity**. Since we learned that genes can 'jump' between viruses and human cells it makes sense that "complex human cells have also developed mechanisms to isolate and fight bacterial and viral invaders, while they wait for the immune system to use adaptive and innate mechanisms.[12]" Cells use a system for recognizing viral DNA sequences[i] and then microRNA's fight back.

In order to infect a cell, bacteria must cross different membranes (remember the cell has an outer membrane, and there are inner membranes too e.g. in mitos. So, in order for the bacteria to get to where they want to go, they must cross multiple membranes and the cell uses clever mechanisms to protect itself with special receptors (**PAMPs** and **DAMPs** (**pathogen and damage associated molecular patterns**) and **PPR** (**pattern recognition receptors**). Don't worry about these names - we will

---

[i]CRISPR system (clustered regularly interspaced short palindromic repeats)

come across them again later when discussing cell signalling. Suffice to say, the cell uses all the means it can to protect itself from invasion including secreting enzymes, producing anti-viral proteins (viperin and tetherin), all to prevent the virus from replicating. If one does enter somehow, it often hitches a ride via cellular vesicles (lysosomes and endosomes). Proteins called **galectins** detect split vesicle contents inside cells and stimulate cell death (**apoptosis**). It's a constant battle between two evolving foes.

Human Leukocyte Antigens (HLAs)

Human Leukocyte Antigens (HLAs) are found on the surface of nearly every cell in the human body. They help the immune system tell the difference between body tissue and foreign substances. They are like a super-regulator of the immune response – above even T-Regs.

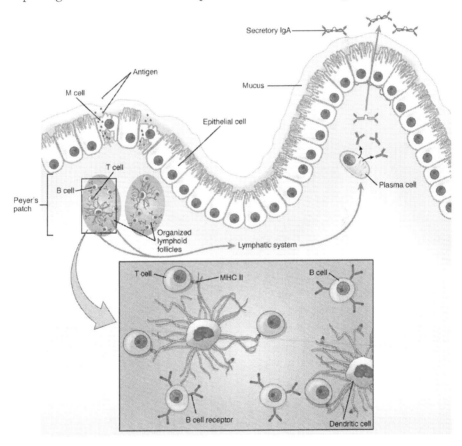

Figure 19: The Gut Associated Lymph Tissue (GALT)

This is a section through the gut lining (epithelial cells shown as little rectangular cells with nuclei). Below this is a dense network of lymphoid tissue which has been magnified for clarity. You can see that the white cells of the immune system (B and T cells) are interspersed between the lymphoid tissues. So, there's very little division between these two systems and constant cellular cross-talk happening. So, anything that helps your lymph to move properly is going to help you maintain good immunity. We can use things like lymphatic drainage massage to help increase the movement of fluids and other different ways to stimulate the lymphatic system: skin brushing, various forms of exercise such as rebounding (trampolining) and walking, infra-red sauna therapy[i], and so on to mobilise the lymphatic system - muscular contraction does that naturally.

There is some important work being done currently that investigates initiation of lymphatic cell growth called **lymphangiogenesis**[13] in cancer which we cover in Chapter 8. But an understanding of lymphatics is important in health too – not least because everything produced by the body passes through either of the vascular (blood) or lymphatic systems.

Autonomic Nervous System

The autonomic nervous system is a very important branch of your central nervous system that controls your body – automatically without conscious control. I went into detail about it in my first book about trauma and survival as it's very implicated in that process.

The autonomic nervous system consists of two branches (and three levels) - the sympathetic and two parasympathetic. They are the upper parasympathetic – rest and digest ventral vagal complex system (VVC-directed by the smart vagus), the sympathetic (fight and flight) and then the **dorsal vagal complex (DVC)** or freeze response[ii] which is a hypo-metabolic survival state which, according to Naviaux, "permits survival and persistence under conditions of environmental stress but at the cost of severely curtailed function and quality of life."[14] This last system is unknown to medical science currently but explains a lot of the features of

---

[i] Infra-red energy mimics the resonant frequency at a cellular level i.e 9.4 microns, helping cells to expel water into the blood and lymphatics and therefore to detoxify. It also marks a shift from sympathetic to parasympathetic activation so is profoundly relaxing. It takes time to work, you have to build up gradually at lower temperatures to encourage sweating,
[ii] Also sometimes called the dauer or hibernation response in animals

chronic illness. Together, these two branches constitute a balanced system which basically control the same organs and tissues but in opposite ways.

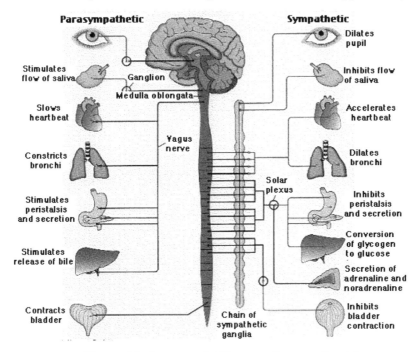

Figure 20: Autonomic Nervous System (basic)

This is important. This means for every function – say bladder control - there is an opposite and balancing reaction. The sympathetic system (fight and flight) closes the bladder sphincter in order to prepare the body for action (and also at night to prepare for sleep interestingly). The parasympathetic (rest and digest) does the opposite. In extreme cases of survival threat – the parasympathetic freeze response – the DVC) will actually enforce defecation and bladder release as you'll have perhaps witnessed in films, etc. People have no conscious control over this and that is the main feature of the autonomic nervous system. It happens quite without conscious control as it integrates with ancient reptilian and mammalian parts of our brain (brainstem and limbic brain) – automatically.

Now, we need to see how this integrates with the cell. The autonomic nervous system runs our physiology. All cells have receptors for the main neurotransmitter **acetylcholine** – the main neurotransmitter of the autonomic nervous system. This opens the cellular membrane gates (transport proteins) for certain enzymes and then genes to be signaled for more specific responses as we've seen. This in turn sends a signal to the rest of the cell via the kinase network to shutdown or stimulate various proteins (structural or functional) then secreted into the cytosol where they produce effects that we may perceive as increase or decrease in energy or ageing. Thus *our symptoms are feedback from this system*. If we then interpret these symptoms in our minds as 'bad', we may get a fear response which further imbalances the system. We need to stimulate the parasympathetic system to rebalance it towards healing.

Neuro-endocrine System and the Heart

One of the most important parts of the system for our discussion is the link between the neurological (nervous) and endocrine (hormone) system. This plays a big part in how we feel – literally, as it happens. The nerves signal to our brain the state of play in our external and internal environments and, with the links to the various **endocrine glands**, they then secrete hormones (chemical messengers) to signal processes like development, sex differentiation, temperature regulation, etc. This coordination of our body's functions is mostly undertaken by the **autonomic nervous system** as shown overleaf.

But chemical messengers are not the only means by which the neuro-endocrine system works. There is also the electromagnetic signalling that glands such as the thyroid and heart produce – the heart has a large electromagnetic signal which is easily measurable. Its purpose is to regulate the brain by producing a signal of coherent waves. The heart has its own nervous system which controls the heart rate in synchrony with the breath.

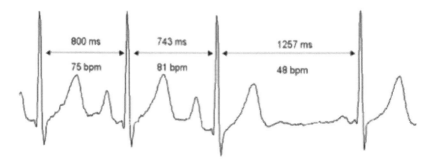

Figure 21: Heart Rate Interval Variation

Note that the interval between heart beats varies – i.e. speeds up when we breathe in (sympathetic activation) and slows down when we breathe out (parasympathetic activation). This is normal and desirable – it's a measure of adaptability and connection between heart and brain. Now, if we measure the *change* in interval between beats and plot that against time, it forms a pattern of sine waves called heart rate variability (HRV). This can be measured simply by measuring blood flow in the finger or arm. This HRV measurement is acutely sensitive to the outside environment. See the diagram overleaf for an output of HRV in a stressed and non-stressed situation. Notice the huge difference – it's a great signal that can be measured as a diagnostic tool.

It is a sign of what is termed 'coherence'. Gregg Braden, author of The Divine Matrix describes it as "harmonizing the heart and the brain through its heart-brain coherence". That this exists as a field that is measurable and can be changed by intention is now no longer the radical notion that it was when he published that book in 2006[15]. In his latest book, Human by Design, he updates that theory with an idea that this is a uniquely human trait given to us, perhaps intentionally, by changes in Chromosome 2 of our 23 pairs[16]. It is an intriguing thought.

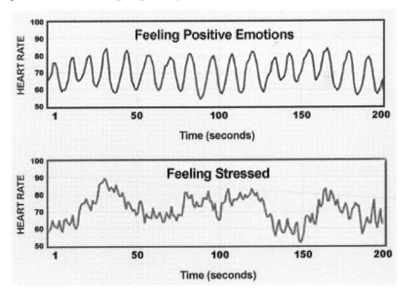

Figure 22: HRV Measurement

It is a most important signal that most doctors are unaware of and simply do not measure – yet it is probably the single most important measure of health and longevity there is. Notice that when feeling stressed[i] the HRV is irregular and jagged; in a harmonious, positive frame the beautiful sine wave (above in the diagram) is seen. In my book The Scar that Won't Heal[17], I talked about it extensively so I won't repeat here but do consider getting one of the many free or low cost apps on smart phones and devices that are now available. Simply type HRV into your search engine to get some examples or contact me for a list which I keep updated as I trial new ones.

Neuropeptides and Cytokines

There is another method of communication which the body uses "to orchestrate many key bodily processes body linking behaviour and biology to effect a smooth functioning of the organism[18]" - small proteins called **neuropeptides**. This network of many different molecules was first described by Candace Pert in her seminal work 'The Molecules of Emotion' and introduced to a new audience via the film 'What the Bleep do we Know?', Candace describes the symphony of different neuropeptides as our 'psychosomatic network' i.e. they link mind and body so that the thoughts we think are translated into these biochemicals.

Primarily considered to be just present in the brain, more recent research has isolated these peptides in the immune system too, where it appears they orchestrate mood[19] and immunity by interaction with other immune cells like T-cell, B-cells and the various **cytokines.** These specialist peptides synthesised by immune cells are considered the 'armed forces' of the immune system and consist of many wonderfully named molecules such as chemokines, interleukins, interferon, **tumour necrosis factor alpha (TNF-α)**, and so on with both pro- and anti- inflammatory actions. Some are even able to permeate the **blood-brain barrier[ii]** and thus affect mood[20] by interaction with the microglial (immune) cells of the brain.[21] We cover that in more detail in the next Chapter.

---

[i] Note stress can be subconscious so not obvious to the person feeling it e.g. you're in a work or relationship situation out of your control which you've got used to but your body responds autonomically anyhow.
[ii] Various theories abound as to how they do this – via the vagus nerve of being 'carried' by various bacteria.

Here is an example of a type of communication system which tells the body exactly how we are feeling in a directly physiological way. It can traverse between brain and body (which was previously thought to be isolated by the BBB). Various theories about how they do this either via a 'Trojan horse' effect with parasites (they traverse inside the parasite or virus) or through **lipid raft signalling** (microdomains of the cell membrane with high lipids that enhance transmission).[22] This has recently been the subject of much research effort to try and enhance drug delivery to the brain[23] (certain phyto-nutrients and microbes do this naturally.). We will return to these in the later chapters on disease but for now just understand that as far as systems biology is concerned, the mind and body are one.

The Body Electric

We are bioelectric beings. The very fact that we can measure the electrical signals of the brain or heart, indicate this fact but it is often forgotten. Another example is that when touched, the skin registers a piezo-electric effect which can be measured.

Importance of the thyroid

The thyroid gland is considered to be an important endocrine gland (the master sex hormone glad) that secretes **thyroxine ($T3^i$)** to control metabolism. This view of the thyroid as 'just another organ' that can malfunction and be removed is so far from the truth. Even the idea that it produces only 4 hormones is, in fact, wrong. There are at least 27 variants that we know of the active T3 hormone called thryomins, thryonins and so on[24]. Their balance is vital.

However, according to recently emerging science of **bioenergetics**, it appears not just to be an endocrine gland but to have an electromagnetic coordinating signal to the rest of the body. It does, interestingly, sit at the junction of mind and body, being situated around the oesophagus in the neck. This is no accident I feel. It helps us to orchestrate our passion, purpose and meaning in the world. Our 'juice' for life, if you will. When our life does not reflect our inner calling, whether because of external threats or internal conflicts, our thyroid will reduce its output to allow us to sink into

---

iSo-called as it has 3 iodines attached. The thyroid concentrates iodine and other elements

a kind of helplessness and despondency that allows us to get through it[i]. It cannot stay that way though if we are to thrive.

Some even consider it the seat of the soul (though few in the conventional medical world will mention the word!). I talked about the importance of the thyroid in my second book 'The World Within' and ideas for recovery from thyroid dysfunction, which is a largely undiagnosed epidemic sweeping Western nations. But in a recent book by Anthony William[25], he postulates that the thyroid is an electromagnetic organ that is being decimated by constant **electromagnetic radiation** (**EMR**) and stress. This would explain the explosion of thyroid disorders, though I feel it is a combination of external and internal factors. According to Dr Berndt Rieger it is also a reflection of how disconnected and competitive our society has become[26].

Electromagnetic Radiation Damage

There is considerable scientific support for the many damaging effects of EMR at a cellular level where it is known that:

"Patho-physiological mechanisms of interaction of EMR at (the) plasma membrane are: calcium efflux from cell membranes, increased expression of stress proteins, influence on channels/gap junctions in cell membranes, overproduction of reactive oxygen species (pro-inflammatory molecule), reduction in melatonin levels, damage to DNA and changes in gene expression in brain cells and an altered blood-brain barrier (BBB)"[27]

Sounds quite bad doesn't it? However, these results are largely shown in tissue samples rather than human beings and we really haven't had these high levels of EMR around very long, so the evidence is still inconclusive on the *long-term effects* of cell-phone interaction, but is likely to have a less than harmonious interaction with our own finely regulated system.

Nerve Conduction

We are electrical beings – something that a lot of people forget. Nerves conduct electricity along the nerve fibre (conductor) which is insulated by **myelin** (insulating sheath); like any electrical wire it needs to protect the signal. Each nerve fibre has many elongated extensions like the branches of

---

[i] Times of life when Hashimotos, a form of auto-immune hypo-thyroiditis, is most likely to strike are for women, puberty, childbirth and then the years of responsibility where for instance we have to take care of others and ignore our own needs and desires.

a tree, which form myriad connections with other nerve fibres and, ultimately, with various organs that the nerve innervates.

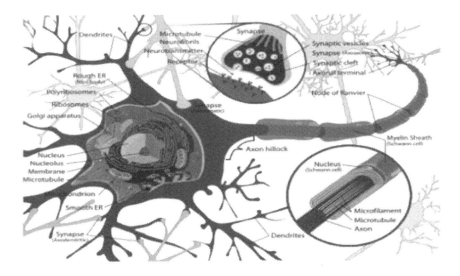

Figure23: Nerve Fibre Structure

At the end of the nerve fibre is a gap called the **synapse** where neurotransmitters like **serotonin, noradrenaline** and **GABA** are secreted to allow the nerve signal (an electrical potential) to 'jump the gap' to link up many different neurons electrochemically.

But as we've already seen in Chapter 1, there is a mismatch between the required speed of human complex movements and the speed of electrical signals (let alone the much slower chemical interactions of hormones) can achieve in the time that we observe them. Some people call this the **credibility gap**. Things like the finely co-ordinated movements of a dancer or concert pianist are hard to explain in electrical or chemical terms – they are simply too slow to produce the wonderful complexity of human movement (not to mention the split second acrobatic turns of birds in flight as seen during a starling murmuration). How then to explain these? Many people believe this is the function of quantum biology, which only operates at very small scales. So we will now turn to an even smaller scale in understanding the cellular nature of humans.

The Brain-Gut-Microbiota Axis

For years we have known that the gut has a neurological network termed 'the gut-brain' (or enteric brain) which possesses vast neuronal connections (100 billion neurons - more than in the spinal cord!). However, we now have to extend this model to include the influence of the microbiota (the sum total of all the microbes that live in and on you) - hence the new term **brain-gut-microbiota axis (BGM)**[28]. This involves elements of the "central nervous system (CNS), the neuro-endocrine and neuro-immune systems, the sympathetic and parasympathetic arms of the **autonomic nervous system (ANS)**, the enteric nervous system – gut nervous system)" and, of course, the microbiome" that colonise us."[16]

This new understanding recognises that *neurological function is highly affected by the state of our microbiome* - a departure from most current teaching in medical schools and how we treat mental illness. The gut and the bacteria in the gut are inextricably and intricately interwoven with brain function. This flies in the face of all we have previously been taught i.e. *that a problem in the brain has its root in the brain* e.g. as in the study of Alzheimer's Disease which has been almost exclusively looking at problems in brain physiology. But we are not making very much progress in controlling or eradicating that disease, in fact it could be said we are losing ground[i]. I would warrant that we are looking in the wrong place as suggested many years ago by the Greek scholar Hippocrates, who said (I paraphrase) "all disease begins in the gut".

Microbiome - human beings as a community of organisms

Our understanding of ourselves has taken an important leap forward in the last decade with the discovery of the amazing diversity of the **microbiome**[ii]. Not just in your gut but on your skin, eyes and even in your brain; microbes constitute the community that lives in and on us. Consisting of around 30 thousand different species of bacteria, 5 million fungi and various other life forms, it constitutes an incredible resource for the manufacture of important hormones, neurotransmitters and enzymes. It has been said that we are not even individual humans but an environment that

---

[i] Rates of all chronic neurological diseases are increasing steadily.
[ii] Strictly speaking, the microbiome is the genetic contribution and microbiota the community themselves but common usage has used the microbiome for both.

bacteria has colonised. There are indeed more microbes than human cells in symbiotic relationship.

We give them warmth and shelter and they help us digest our food, control immunity and brain function. This community of gut and skin bacteria – your microbiome – is key to your health and wellbeing. When they are in good balance with a high diversity, you are likely to be healthy. Their interaction with the cells of our gut lining helps prime the immune system and the products of their metabolism are vital for us. They make a large proportion of the brain neurotransmitters we need e.g. 70-90% of serotonin (happy), GABA (calm, balanced), dopamine (motivation, drive) and acetylcholine (memory) and are made in the gut by microbes for instance.

Remember neurotransmitters are neuro-chemicals that allow neurons (nerve cells) to synapse (join electrochemically) and communicate with each other. If most of our neurotransmitters are made in the gut, then if the gut is out of balance, so will be all our neurotransmitters and thus our neurological function will be compromised[i]. Not only that, but our first-line immune defence system lines the gut – called the **innate immune system**. It learns what is friend or foe from the signals propagated by microbial balance. So if the balance is wrong, the potential for faulty recognition of 'self' and auto-immune attack is much more likely.

Microbial RNA Sequencing

Recently scientists have been looking at **RNA sequencing** of stool samples of a large number of people in order to determine the commonalities and patterns. Remember RNA is the copy that is made of DNA before making proteins. A large proportion in the gut comes from microbes (perhaps 100:1). The RNA produced is called the expression or **phenotype** of our genes (DNA **genotype**) and shows you what microbes are present and what they are doing. By comparing large numbers of people they are able to generate a data-set showing microbial RNA and matching that to certain disease states compared to healthy guts. Scientists can then build computer models (via artificial intelligence (AI)) to explore what might happen when you have certain combinations i.e. develop a *predictive* capability. RNA

---

[i]Dr DatisKharrazianbelieves in fact that we can work out where we are inflamed by the type of function that is compromised e.g if our balance is poor then our cerebellum is compromised.

activity is a better judge of what's actually going on as it is further downstream of the process of reading the genes

Gene (DNA) $\rightarrow$ RNA $\rightarrow$ proteins

transcription translation

Analysis of the microbial RNA shows which new microbes are transient (trespassers) and which have become resident. It is then possible to make recommendations of supplementation based on the data sample across the population rather than individuals.

But be aware it's not as simple as just taking **probiotics** to supplement the deficiencies. Recent research has cast doubt on this approach as it tends to take longer to re-balance the gut than if it was left to itself (and certainly longer than if you ate specific probiotic foods to encourage certain microbes)[29]. Food is always better than supplements but of course finding healthy bacterial-rich food is difficult in today's sterile world.

The quickest way to restore a good microbiome is to inoculate with the faeces of a healthy person – this is called a **faecal microbiome transplant (FMT)**. Believe it or not, despite the yuck factor, this approach is gaining ground in conventional medicine as a way to reverse many chronic disease states! This is generally done in clinical situations and with people who have come to the end of the road with conventional approaches. It might one day become the conventional approach, who knows!

When we understand that this microbially integrated system is highly influenced by the body's cellular chemistry, we can look to what controls this; primarily our nutrition and lifestyle which either promotes or reduces inflammation in the body[i]. So, we need to address what David Perlmutter, expert in brain physiology, calls, "root-cause resolution practices." In other words, we need to look beyond the organ that is having the issue and turn to altering the systemic (whole body) up-regulation of inflammation.

Dietary practice is the main influence which triggers inflammatory cascades throughout the BGM. The permeability of the gut lining (aka 'leaky gut') is a cardinal player in this cascade. There are several factors that increase gut

---

[i] Although a good inflammatory response is part of the body's attempt to destroy pathogens and thus essential for survival , it can rapidly accelerate the aging process if it becomes chronic

permeability. Gluten is one of the main players (via the **zonulin** mechanism which opens up the junctions between cells). However, even without permeability, just gut dysbiosis (imbalance of gut flora) can still give us inflammation. The microbes that line the gut sit on the lining cells or epithelium and it's only one cell thick.

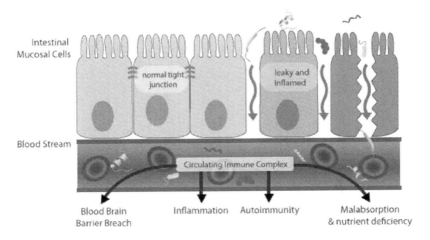

Figure 24: Gut Permeability aka 'Leaky Gut'

So now we know that adding probiotics to the diet as a 'quick fix' has been discounted; as most orally administered probiotics are just transient and don't take up permanent residence in the gut. Indeed most probiotics tablets aren't even based on what should be there but on what is cheap to produce commercially! This normally correlates to what can be found in the gut of cows as they are easy to propagate and produce for sale in bulk. So you'll notice a lot of Lactobacillus and Bifidobacterium which are not necessarily what you need.

Clearly creating a healthy brain-gut-microbiome is not about pill popping, whether pharmaceutical or nutritional supplements. It is more sophisticated and variable – depending on that individual person and the environment they are in. In the next chapter I will be looking at how these systems are co-ordinated, particularly in light of threats to the smooth running of these networks.

Chapter 3: Perturbations of the System

Now that I have described the biological systems that are subject to environmental influence, and the ageing process, I need to consider how we exchange information with our environment: the natural and unnatural modifications to the system. Some are natural, some man-made – we will discuss each of these in turn and then consider how they impact the normal functions of the body.

Genes are not your Destiny: Epigenetics

There is another layer to the story of genetic regulation which has been coined **epigenetics**- which means 'above genetics'. This is the next layer of complexity, as it helps determine which genes are expressed. This is a complete paradigm shift in our understanding of human complexity and it goes some way to explaining why it is we have so few genes, compared to prior predictions based on our observed complexity.

Remember, we have barely any more genes than a worm (some now estimate we have less!) The number of human genes keeps being revised downwards as we work out the function of the non-coding DNA. The current figure of 20,000 genes is certainly not enough to explain how we came to be so much more complex. Clearly there is something missing in this 'genetic determinism' understanding i.e. that everything in life is determined by the random endowment of genetic information from our parents. Indeed, the discovery of epigenetics shows us that it is not just the genes but *how they are read* that determines how well we live and age. In short, this means certain 'environmental factors' turn the genes on and off in a complex orchestration between groups of genes. Much like the words in a sentence can be combined in a multitude of ways, the genes plus environment create different *expressions*. That expression changes in response to the signals it receives internally and externally – it is a real-time readout.

So what are the epigenetic factors that control this readout? Recent discoveries have highlighted some unexpected contributors: firstly the microbes in your gut, on your skin, etc contribute their own DNA – collectively called the microbiome. Microbes are well known for their ability to multiply and adapt much more quickly than we can. Their DNA interacting with ours gives us a much more responsive mechanism to adapt or compensate to subtle changes in the environment.

Epigenetic Mechanisms

So, what is the mechanism that allows environmental influences to change the readout? It's important to understand that DNA doesn't just float around in the cell at random – it is tightly contained within the chromosomes by being wound around like a ball of twine[i]. This is to protect it from being damaged – to be 'read', sections of it must be carefully unwound. There are various ways in which the *readability* of the DNA can be changed: by adding chemical (acetyl or methyl groups[ii]) to control the way the DNA is wrapped and unwrapped via proteins called **histones**. It's like adding highlights to the blueprint that say 'ignore this bit' or 'use this'. It helps explain the conundrum as to how a liver cell has the same genetic instructions as a brain cell but very different structure and functions. How does the cell know which ones to read and which ones to ignore?

"Even though every cell in your body starts off with the same DNA sequence, give or take a couple of letters here and there, the text has different patterns of highlighting in different types of cell - a liver cell doesn't need to follow the same parts of the instruction manual as a brain cell. But the really interesting thing about epigenetics is that the marks aren't fixed in the same way the DNA sequence is: some of them can change throughout your lifetime, and in response to outside influences. Some can even be inherited, just like some highlighting still shows up when text is photocopied."[30]

The important point about these environmental epigenetic regulators is that they can *adapt much more quickly than genetic changes* are able to. Hence if the body needs to shut down energy quickly to save itself, it is able to do so

---

[i] There is on average about 6ft of DNA per cell i.e. a lot compared to the size of the cell!
[ii] Acetyl groups unwrap and methyl groups wrap the section of DNA to allow or prevent access to the genes being read or 'transcribed'

without waiting for the inevitable time lag it takes to read the DNA and create new proteins. This is a reason that many people are suffering from chronic (long-term) diseases as the constant flow of epigenetic factors towards energy conservation and survival of the whole is prioritised over relaxation, creativity and health. These activities are not deemed important enough for overall survival so are shut down.

Since we now know that some of these epigenetic changes are *heritable* (we inherit the epigenetic mechanisms as well as the genetic code), it begins to seem a plausible explanation for why some trauma passes down the generations in the form of susceptibility to stress and long-term health issues[ii]. Through this lens we see that disease is not random, but an *inevitable result of altered biochemistry to perceived threat* and thus it destroys the current medical model of baffling, random, unconnected symptoms.

Indeed Dr Jeffrey Bland, dubbed the 'father of functional medicine' has suggested that "the idea that multiple diseases co-existing independently from one another (in the same patient) is being replaced by the understanding that the origins of illness can be traced to the same physiological disturbances and common underlying pathways"[31]. Thus his theory is that diseases are a 'delusion' of the human mind and its wish to classify, borne of the origins of medicine in treating largely infectious diseases where there was *a specific pathogen which caused the same disease in all people* e.g. tuberculosis by the bacterium, Mycobacterium tuberculosis.

In this new medical model we redefine the disease process as *a natural result of imbalance in the system* – a systems approach to health and wellbeing called **systems biology**[iii]. Holistic medicine (functional/natural medicine) comes closest to this understanding and deals with the resulting 'disease' very differently. When we look 'upstream', the causes of diseases are the same: disruptions to cell health and gene expression. According to cardiologist Dr Mark Houston "there are infinite assaults on the vascular system but only 3

---

[i] Most of the experimental evidence for this is in mice rather than humans; but it has been observed in the children and grandchildren of Holocaust survivors and those subjected to the Dutch 'Hunger Winter' during WWII for instance.

[ii] So-called intergenerational trauma – very common in people with chronic illness for instance, is the trauma not only of their childhood's but their parents (and sometimes grandparents!).

[iii] It borrows its ideas from engineering but applied to the body

responses: inflammation, oxidative stress and immune dysfunction"[32]. We can generalise this to the body as a whole.

Our environment has changed rapidly in the last 60 years or so, more rapidly than at any point in our history. There are more toxins, stress, poor quality food, disconnection with the earth and its seasons and so on, which mean we are getting discordant messages which the body struggles to cope with. Of all the messages, that which we take directly into our bodies, food, is the biggest epigenetic modifier of all (though stress comes a close second). "The human genome and the epigenetic expression of that genome are based on what it learned thousands of years ago from whole, natural foods. Eventually science will prove that refined sugar and partially-hydrogenated vegetable oils are the leading health destroyers of our times as both are highly inflammatory at the cell membranes — (both) cell wall and mitochondrial."[33]. Unfortunately, because of our focus on profit over health in food manufacture, these two cheap substances are primary ingredients in our diets today and cholesterol is denigrated instead.

According to Dr Natasha Campbell McBride, an expert in dietary management of disease, "when you attack cholesterol, you are 'attacking the ambulance and not the problem'". As I described in my last book:

"Cholesterol is in fact an essential molecule in the body[34]; an important component of the cell membrane, keeping it flexible and thus allowing it to interact with its neighbours[i]. But it has been unfairly demonised as the enemy, largely because it is extremely profitable to promote the 'high cholesterol causes heart disease myth' as it sells profitable statin drugs".

The Epigenome

Both our native cells and those of the microbiome are regulated by the **epigenome** (the multitude of chemicals that regulate the genome); they are one unit. Genetic expression can be influenced by nutrients, toxins and even thoughts and feelings which trigger the stress response and immune systems. When they are overtly negative, they can become fixed in a habitual pattern of threat to the system which can even be transmitted to the next generation. Even the way we are conceived seems to have epigenetic consequences; "a process called epigenetic imprinting adjusts the

---

[i] The cell membrane is an electrochemical transducer, allowing messages in and out.

54

activity of genes that will shape the character of the child yet to be conceived."[35] Whether this is solely by epigenetics or by behavioural influences is a moot point; it probably involves both. What is undisputed is that we can influence our children and their children by the way we lead our lives and take care of our relationship to ourselves'.

The implications of this realisation for our interaction with our microbiome are *huge*. If 2.2m genes come from microbiome compared to 20,000 from our own, then *99% of the DNA in our bodies is microbial.* Just think of the multitude of epigenetic fine tuning that is possible with this amount of extra DNA, RNA and protein interactions. Without these microbes, you would be unable to speak a sentence, or think, let alone digest your food. This intimate interaction regulates our functioning more than our own genes so getting the balance of flora right and respecting their input into our evolutionary history is vital. We have co-evolved with the microbes so every cell in your body has the entire history of evolution in those genes.[73] As Deepak Chopra has said, "your ancestors are alive in you!" Once we realise we are constantly passing on epigenetic modulations onto our genes, we are encouraged to take better care of our cellular environment.

Stress and the Cell

Stress is endemic and, according to Dr Jeffrey Thompson, 'the ultimate epigenetic determinant'; specifically the unresolved beliefs, emotions and behaviours programmed subconsciously from early life experience, inescapable circumstances in our relationships, work-life and so on, and chemical and environmental stress of toxins, poor food and uncontrolled exposure to electromagnetic radiation (EMR). Stress becomes a chronic feature of our lives under these circumstances and our autonomic nervous system is thus permanently switched to a state of readiness for attack; a so-called **sympathetic dominance** or **'fight and flight'** state.

He has found by measuring heart rate variability (HRV) of a sample of people that most peoples' stress response is constantly switched on, even when they lie down to go to sleep! This prevents us from healing overnight at a cellular level; the brainwaves seldom go into their slowest frequency range called theta – 1.5 Hz which is the healing state. Certain techniques like meditation and binaural beats[i] (asynchronous auditory recordings of

---

[i] Also sometimes called holosync – the names vary depending on who developed it.

different frequency played into each ear), claim to re-train the brain to do this.

In the past we would have used sound, light and grounding with the earth and its rhythms to do this. Dr Thompson and others aren't making a claim for a return to some idealised ancient world (although it would be good if we got more connected to nature), but about harnessing modern technology to return us to our optimum state as programmed into our neurology for hundreds of thousands of years. It's an exciting time to be alive when we realise we can overcome our human limitations.

Cellular Stress Response

Stress is anything that shifts the body outside of its normal range of physiological balance or *homeostasis*. Light amounts of stress are good for us – they induce a state of **hormesis** or rejuvenation – particularly important to keep your mitochondria fit and healthy with frequent turnover. However, if stress is chronic and unrelenting, too much adrenaline and cortisol (the stress hormones) damage the mitochondria by interfering with their signalling, and they start to get overwhelmed. So, mild stress or reduced nutrients tends to enhance oxidative phosphorylation (oxphos - the form of efficient energy production), whereas too much stress, excess nutrients, disease and inflammation, induces mitochondrial fission (separation) and **mitophagy** (destruction) and reduced oxphos making us sick. The exception is cancer where uncontrolled growth may result from loss of natural cell destruction.

So, when people have more stress than their bodies can handle (and that includes poor food, sedentary, isolated lives and unresolved emotions or shame-driven beliefs), their mitochondrial functioning is severely impaired. Many people are now coming round to the idea that Chronic Fatigue Syndrome (CFS) and cancer are primarily mitochondrial disorders but the list may include most chronic disease to some extent.

As soon as there is some stress on the body, the body generates superoxide free radicals which activate the master regulator in the inflammatory pathway: a protein called **NFkB** which controls transcription of DNA, cytokine production and cell survival. The oxidative stress master regulator is a similar protein called NRF2 and they are important as they control all the other genes and downstream pathways. This new way of looking at disease not as an entity but *as a symptom of cellular dysfunction* with the same physiological drivers in operation has opened up a new field of **nutrigenomics,** which looks at the influence of nutrients on gene expression. We will come to this towards the end of this Chapter but first we must consider what else happens in the cell to change its function.

Cell Damage and AGEs

Cells are vulnerable to many different insults as we now see. Infection or invasion by foreign microbes (viruses, bacteria, etc) is another stress the body has to engage with. Up to now we only considered the innate immune system as our first line defence system. But it is becoming clear that the first line of cellular defence is not the specialized immune cells, but is the *individual cell itself.* This surprising ability of cells, called **cell autonomous immunity**, shows that non-immune cells also combat microbes. This is a new area of research that is very promising.

There is one type of molecule, however, particularly involved with ageing of the cell. **Advanced glycation end products (AGEs)** are formed where sugars become attached to proteins (a process called **glycation**). They are a serious problem as far as the body is concerned as they change the structure and function of the protein and the body can no longer recognize them as native proteins. They are then marked as foreign and the body mounts an immune attack against them.

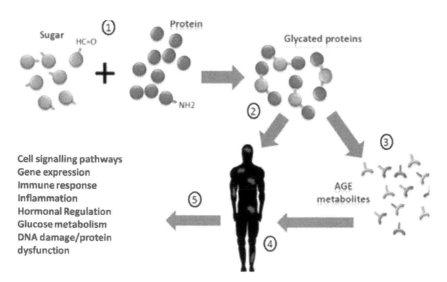

Figure 25: AGEs and Health

How do AGEs form? There are two routes: one is ingestion of food, the other is production by the body itself (including our resident microbiota). They profoundly impact our health and wellbeing, as protein function depends largely on its 3-dimensional structure in space. You may have come across health advice, heavily promoted in the media very recently, to avoid chargrilled meats[i] and other highly processed food produce. Why so? Well cooking protein at high temperatures causes glycation resulting in AGEs or 'crusty protein[ii]' as Jeffrey Bland calls them[36]. These products in food are bad news for our health – they promote cellular **inflammation**, the basis of all disease.

AGEs induce pathology not just by the formation of crosslinked proteins, (thus directly altering their structure and therefore their function). They also activate intracellular signals through several receptor- and nonreceptor-mediated mechanisms, leading to an increased production of reactive oxygen species and inflammatory cytokines. One of the best-studied AGE receptors is RAGE (no prizes for guessing what that stands for).

---

[i] It's called the Maillard reaction and animal foods cooked at a high temperature for a prolonged period of time and under dry conditions will have the highest AGE content
[ii] It's the same process as when a crust forms on bread in a hot oven – tasty but damaged.

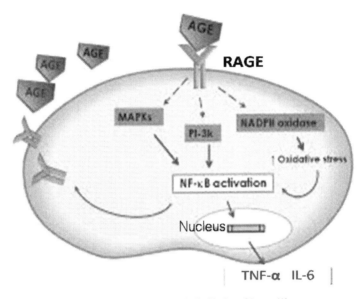

Figure 26: AGES and Cellular Signalling

In addition they "play an important role in the pathogenesis of diabetic complications"[37] in particular and are the cause of skin ageing,[38] especially liver spots on the hands and face. With sunshine exposure the AGEs go dark brown/black, but, more worryingly, they are linked to ageing of blood vessels with heart disease implications.

But they also form naturally in the body *without heat* when blood sugar (**glucose**) reacts with **haemoglobin A1c (HbA1c)** protein, a naturally occurring AGE in the blood (within red blood cells). It is routinely used as a measure of blood glucose when monitoring diabetes. The average lifespan of a red blood cell is 120 days so not such an issue as with many other proteins in the skin and blood vessels. According to recent research it "may be particularly important in the context of long-lived proteins that do not undergo rapid synthesis and turnover"[39]. This would include proteins involved in nerve signal transmission for instance which may explain the damaged proteins observed in many neurodegenerative conditions.

Cell Defence: Heat Shock Response, DAMPs and PAMPs

Another response of the cell to damage comes after injury or stress such that the cell organelles (mitochondria and others) release small fragments of the damaged organelle as *signalling molecules*. These are termed damage associated molecular patterns (DAMPs) which include uric acid, ATP, heat shock proteins and hyaluronic acid (which we have met already). A similar thing happens when a bacterium is broken down by the immune system to form pathogen associated molecular proteins (PAMPs). Remember mitochondria are simply bacteria that came to live with us permanently through evolution and they share many of the same structure and survival mechanisms[i].

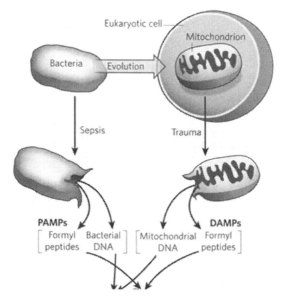

Figure 27: Cell Defence - Heat Shock Response

The ATP and proteins released from both these processes (DAMPs and PAMPs) combine to produce the **heat shock response.** This is of particular interest as it consists of the formation of certain endogenous cellular protein protectors called **heat shock proteins (HSPs).**

When under stress, the cell must do more to keep its proteins from being denatured (the 3-D shape or conformation changed) so it releases a DNA transcription (reading) molecule called **heat shock factor (HSF).** Unbound HSF is normally inactive and floating in the cytoplasm where it can begin to

---

[i] And give us of course immense epigenetic variance and adaptability of response as well as a very efficient means of respiration (energy production)

aggregate and cause damage. When a stress occurs, chaperone proteins bind to the HSF and cause it to move to the nucleus and bind with other HSF into groups of three – termed **trimerisation** which activates it. This trimer HSF then binds to heat shock elements (HSE) on the DNA to activate transcription (production) of messenger RNA (mRNA). The mRNA will eventually make more HSPs that can alleviate the stress at hand and restore homeostasis "The activation of this pathway is a primary defence mechanism that protects cells from stress conditions that promote protein misfolding, aggregation and cell death.[40]"

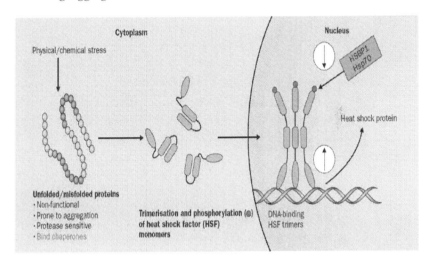

Figure 28: Heat Shock Response

By helping to 'chaperone' other native proteins inside the cell, they enable the cell to withstand insults like the sudden increase in oxygen requirement of exercise, oxidative stress and **hypoxia** (low oxygen). Proteins are very dependent on their three dimensional shape – needing to be folded in a certain way to perform their functions well. When subject to damage, proteins no longer function and will need to be recycled or repaired. HSP's are part of that cyto-protective response system. So HSP's help bind to misfolded proteins and chaperone them into the cell and then to the nucleus where they produce more adaptive proteins. Relevant to our discussion is that neurons interchange HSP's with their 'helper' glial cells to protect the neuron from oxidative stress. So they are part of the cell protection response.

Certain foods are known to induce the production of various different HSP's (which are numbered according to their molecular weight). For instance, **resveratrol**, a plant compound found in red wine, is known to induce expression of various HSP's and, in particular to inhibit, HSP27 and HSP70 in human tumour cells. We will return to the importance of foods as an epigenetic modifier in cancer in Chapter 8. Certainly, HSP's are starting to be seen as a hidden reason why certain diets are good for us.

The Cell Danger Response

If these disrupted messages go on for long enough, the cell beings to operate under an alarm state known as the **Cell Danger Response (CDR)**. This has been highlighted by the work of the cell biologist Dr. Robert Naviaux, who showed that the messengers of the cellular environment are highly implicated as I described in my first book:

"mitochondria are intelligent, dynamic organelles which can respond to the environment. When the cell senses a threat, it activates the Cell Danger Response (CDR), aerobic (oxygen-using) respiration is down-regulated and our cells shift to the alternative pathway outside the mitochondria which, as we saw earlier is anaerobic and produces much less ATP from glucose (the sugar that we burn). This means less energy is available for all the work of the cell; repair, renewal, cell signalling and protein manufacture. The cell goes on a 'go slow' and if the CDR does not abate, the cell becomes fixed in this pattern which is highly dangerous for the organism (us)."

Remember in the previous chapter we looked at the communication structure that all cells are bathed in called the ECM? This is the informational matrix that transmits the messages of the cell to the rest of the body. Changes to this matrix during the CDR include certain damage associated molecular patterns, heat shock proteins and different proteins that modulate the opening and closing of the mitochondrial membrane so that *energy is conserved to prioritise survival over quality of life.*

They are highly conserved evolutionary processes that are integral in the protection against perceived threat. Before the adaptive or even the innate immune system responds to threat, the cells and particularly the signals that occur within the mitochondria sense that there has been a threat to the particular cell in question. This begins a series of events that takes place that alters the metabolism of the cell; down-regulating from fourth gear to second gear, shutting methylation down along with consumption of energy via ATP, to begin a co-ordinated *defence program* initiated by the mitochondria. And this initiates a co-ordinated cycle of further events. So the ATP gets ejected out of the cell into the extracellular or peri-cellular environment, leading to a number of additional processes including the recruitment of the innate immune system. And it's not just ATP that's involved.

Dr Naviaux used a technique called **metabolomics:** he profiled the fate of 500 metabolites in the cell to plot particular patterns and correlate them to specific disease states. His team postulated and then corroborated that it is activation and the binding of **purinergic receptors** i.e. 'purinergic signalling', which largely signal the cell danger response. Purines are molecules like ATP (the classic energy molecule) but also other molecules too like ADP, UDP; these purines get thrown out of the cell into the peri-cellular (surrounding the cell) space and begin coordinating different inflammatory events. These extracellular nucleotides can then bind to different purinergic receptors and essentially perpetuate the inflammatory cell danger response throughout the tissue and beyond.

Purinergic receptors are the most common receptor type in the human physiology; they are abundant in every tissue type and virtually every cell type, including the central nervous system. They're essential for neural development and for growth and maturation. Their activation in certain cell types activates the mTOR system which we came across in Chapter 1. This stimulates an **anabolic** (building) growth process. Purinergic signalling is at the heart of a co-ordinated cellular growth processes so is vital for normal function.

However, it's recently become clear that *danger signalling* is also highly reliant on these same purinergic systems and certain purine receptors like the P2X and the P2Y receptors perpetuate cell danger signalling. Cells have thus evolved a highly sophisticated mechanism to protect themselves with a complex set of co-ordinated signals (on and off) to regulate this. The problem is that for some people this cell danger signalling *does not switch off* and it perpetuates or contributes greatly to a disease process. What is meant to turn on transiently in the context of some kind of clear threat, whether toxic exposure or an infection or a trauma or suchlike, is then meant to be extinguished. But in some people it seems to stay switched on resulting in chronic inflammatory illness and we need to understand why that is. It's highly likely that this goes back to our **biochemical individuality** from our epigenetic variation where we are interacting differently with our environment to switch certain genes on and off. If the genes for a protein which is meant to attenuate (stop) the CDR is switched off then the CDR will continue unabated. This seems to be what happens in the majority of chronic disease states.

Role of Mitochondria

Navaiux's particular interest is the role of the mitochondria as directors of this process. Don't forget mitochondria reflect our ancestral origins when a proteo-bacterium (early single-celled organism) first fused with a eukaryotic (complex - nucleated) cell, and over time started to co-operate with the cell such that it became part of it. These became the mitochondria that we now think of as part of our own cells but their structure and function give away their bacterial origins. Of course over millennia they have evolved further. They have subsequently specialised to become the main powerhouse and coordinators of the cell and therefore the organism.

So how does this relate to the ECM specifically? Well, part of the CDR process involves the breakdown of **hyaluronic acid (HA)**. This is one of the four major glycoproteins called glycosaminoglycans (GAGs) present in connective tissue (fascia) that provide a number of important functions. For example, in its normal state it is integral for the *hydration of the tissue;* it helps to draw water or biological electrolyte solution into connective tissue. Hyaluronic acid also provides a certain degree of stability and stabilisation to the connective tensile strength just like the other GAGs do. It most likely is involved in electrochemical communication through ionic and water balance mechanisms; something we discussed earlier in the chapter.

When the CDR process causes the breakdown of hyaluronic acid, those HA fragments signal damage-associated molecular protein fragments or DAMPs that are recognised by certain enzymes called metalloproteinases

(MMP's) to break down the matrix further by boring further holes in the system so that the immune cells can penetrate. It's a degenerative process.

Moreover, **mast cells** (a type of immune cell) in the ECM receive the products of this degradation (the purines and extracellular ATP) which then bind to the receptors of the mast cells causing them to degranulate i.e. burst, whereupon they release their contents – mainly histamine. Thus begins the effects of **histamine intolerance** and inflammation. It is worth considering the ECM as an *organ system* that is in dynamic communication with the rest of the organism.

So when you have matrix dys-regulation it has a systemic effect throughout the body. For instance it will affect the hypothalamus in the brain which picks up signals from the body to signal hormonally via the **HPA** and **HPT (Hypothalamus Pituitary Adrenal and Thyroid)** axes. Other factors which deeply affect the ECM are the degree of hydration and light exposure. It is understood that near infrared light increases collagen synthesis so this can be a useful intervention with the use of infra-red light bulbs and saunas. The ECM is involved also as the substrate for the conversion of vitamin D (calcitriol) into an inactive metabolite. This has a direct effect on collagen synthesis in the fibroblasts as well as the change in hormonal synthesis. It's a nicely co-ordinated system until disrupted.

Cellular Detoxification

Next we turn to the response of the cell to toxins of various forms from both within and without.

Cytochrome P450 system

Toxins may come from many sources: they may be environmental or they may be produced naturally as the by-products of normal cellular processes. Our bodies have a system that deals with this and it's called the **cytochrome P450 system (CYP450)** – a series of over 50 enzymes that process and detoxify all manner of molecules to render them harmless. The CYP450 super system exists in the liver (the main organ of detoxification) and generally operates at night when you are asleep. But people are very variable in detoxification ability due to genetic differences – I covered this in much more detail in my first book. Also we are subject to such a deluge of toxins, new environmental chemicals that our systems can become overwhelmed. So the old argument that the body can manage detoxification on its own without any support or promotion is no longer valid[i].

Food as information - Nutrigenomics

Food is more than calories: it is *information*. And the way that information is conveyed is not just in the chemical constituents of our food but its energetic characteristics. Good food is one of the foundations of health so let's look at it in some detail.

In my previous book, I dealt in detail with how you can change your health by manipulating the gut flora via eating different types of food in certain ways. I likened it to 'creating a healthy inner garden' by reducing/cutting out refined carbohydrates and sugars, excess meat and damaged processed fats; all of which imbalance our flora. A lot of the benefits of food are beyond the chemical macronutrients:

"Fresh food, provided it is grown in good soil with access to light and clean air and water, not only gives us the nutrients we need to survive but it also delivers the beneficial bacteria in the correct formulation via its connection with the microbiome of the soil. These microbes then help us create the nutrients we can't make ourselves (or in sufficient number) to be healthy.

The type of food is key: anything that creates systemic inflammation will undoubtedly create poor health outcomes. This includes sugar, dairy and gluten for most people. Sugar is particularly bad, not just because of its addictive qualities and high calorific value; it also combines with the proteins (and some lipids) on the surface of every cell to produce Advanced Glycation End (AGE) products, as we've seen.

Dietary modifications

Two ideas that have become popular recently in modifying our epigenetic responses are fasting and **ketogenesis** (the production of ketones). Fasting need not be a formal period of deliberately not eating, it can simply be expanding your 'fasting window' i.e. the time between your last meal at night and the first meal in the morning. Ever wondered why breakfast was

---

[i] You'll hear this many times from medical doctors and some researchers who believe the detox business is hokum. They may be right about some of the detox remedies but not the necessity for intervention to help detoxification as the huge rise in cancers attests.

called break-fast? Now you know. It's actually incredibly important to not eat late at night as it helps the liver to do its detoxification work overnight without being overburdened.

Ketogenic ('keto') diets are also all the rage at the moment; based on restricting carbohydrates and increasing fats. When you change your diet like this, the body is forced into **ketosis** where it uses fats for energy. The body then converts fats to **ketones**[i] in the liver, which are subsequently transported to the brain where they are used preferentially. The benefit is that fats are a lot less inflammatory than carbs (one of the main reason we have a catastrophic rise in all chronic diseases is our glyphosate-laden, processed carb-heavy diet). However, you need to have a healthy functioning bile to digest fats well and if your liver is struggling you will need liver support to adapt to a keto diet well.

The ideal **fasting window** (length of time between eating your last meal of the day and your first the next day) for ketosis is 12 hours – 15 hours although you would need to avoid carbs completely for 36 hours for full ketosis. You'll notice a characteristic 'sweet' breath odour caused by acetone, although you can buy devices which will measure it in the breath if you're not sure. Ketosis generates substantial health benefits including lowering blood cholesterol and encouraging weight loss – it is known to reduce your likelihood of many of the most common diet-related diseases like heart disease and cancer, as well as the neurological conditions like Alzheimer's and depression.

However it is not for everyone – it can be hard to achieve for some, and there is much machismo on the internet around this – body builders and athletic males competing with each other for how often and how easily they accomplish ketosis. Remember we are all biochemically individual and women and men are very different. too. So, if you are going to experiment with a keto diet get some advice from someone like you (similar age, gender, condition etc) who has done it[ii]. Better still follow a proper diet with a nutritional therapist or functional medicine doctor. Some people

---

[i] One of the most important
[ii] I speak with experience here. I know of a few women who have succeeded in a keto diet – but not many. Women need more carbs than men generally – so other approaches may be better for them.

really struggle going into ketosis so will initially feel much worse (especially if their liver is compromised as I've already said.

So what are other ways we can improve our diets specifically? Here we need to turn to nutrients as they are one way the body takes in information which changes gene expression in real time i.e. epigenetically. Certain nutrients (minerals and vitamins, organic compounds) do this more than others and are therefore considered *essential* to metabolic function. Most are derived from plants and therefore a plant-based (i.e. Mediterranean) diet is the baseline for all of us regardless of our individual preferences. However, we need to be aware that certain molecular components of plants are particularly powerful and it is to this I now turn.

Phyto (Plant-Derived) Nutrients

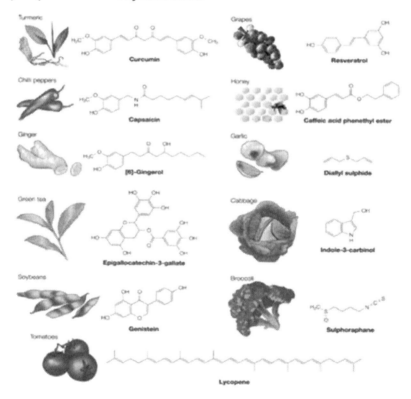

Figure 29: Phyto-nutrients

Since we co-evolved with plants (albeit they've been around a lot longer), it's no surprise that we should have developed a need for certain plant-derived nutrients (**phyto-nutrient**s) e.g. **carotenoids** (like beta-carotene converted to Vitamin A), **lycopene** (in tomatoes), **lutein** and **xanthins** (essential for eye health , **resveratrol** (in red wine and grapes), and even **chlorophyll** itself. They have long been known to have chemical properties that benefit us. However, now that we know a little more about the energetic qualities of these molecules we can describe their benefits more fully as being light frequency based. All are **chromophores**; defined as a natural compound, high in double bonds which resonate (vibrate) at high frequencies in the body absorbing and reflecting light; these are responsible for the bright colour of the food.

The electron transport chain (ETC) in mitochondria contains many different chromophores as part of the chain which facilitates the production of energy within that system. They enable electron and photon (light particle) exchange within the system.[41] Chlorophyll, the plant pigment that makes plants green, is not only used by plants in their energy production as we previously believed. It is also important in increasing the efficiency of animal energy generation by allowing more energy to be produced *without increasing oxidative stress*. Chlorophyll thus makes energy production more efficient and less damaging to the body by reducing free radical (ROS) production (the natural consequence of energy production). Some of the coloured compounds in fruits such as blueberries, strawberries (which contain fisetin) also protect our immune system via **regulatory T-cells (T-regs** - the directors of the immune cell 'army'). Another reason to make sure you eat a 'rainbow diet' with its high levels of these compounds.

Glandulars and Protomorphogens

There is another level of complexity to supplementation which not a lot of people are aware of. For many years we used animal glandulars (ground up animal glands) to treat the common diseases such as thyroid disorders. But since the dominant model of pharmaceutical medicine introduced on the 1950's/60's these more natural remedies became derided and discontinued. They were considered 'unscientific' (an idea promoted by the pharmaceutical industry) and have largely been replaced with synthetic alternatives such as 'Synthroid' for thyroid disease. The problem is these synthetics are composed of just one hormone (in fact the inactive form that needs conversion in the body – T4) and contain none of the complexity of the gland itself. Many people can't convert the synthetic T4 to the active hormone (T3) their body needs[i], or in situations of high inflammation, their body converts it to a deliberately inactive form (**reverse T3 - rT3**) so their body is still struggling despite high levels of T4.

An alternative approach, largely ignored by the scientific establishment (except veterinary medicine interestingly) is the use of **protomorphogens (PMs)**. These are 'tissue-specific protein extracts' first described by Dr Royal Lee:

"who was an early pioneer in human nutrition (and) proposed that glands and organ tissue could be effective beyond their unique vitamin and mineral content. He believed that animal extracts supported cellular health at the level of the nucleus, and in an unbalanced system these extracts could activate cells to repair. In 1947, six years before Watson and Crick defined DNA and the double helix, Dr. Lee proposed his theory of Protomorphology. (which described them) to be the smallest functional units of the chromosome - cell-specific nucleoproteins that provided the blueprint and framework upon which a cell was constructed."[42]

Unfortunately, he was vilified as most innovators are, and today his theories are largely ignored by medicine. Most people have never come across these compounds and there are only a few studies on their use in humans. But they have a good basis in veterinary and naturopathic care and are promoted by companies like Standard Process in the US.

Lee based his studies on the work he did with animals, who often consume the glands and organs of other animals when they eat them. This means the predator appropriates the components of those glands and organs into their own and it is key to health. Unfortunately for us and our pets, this is often not the case now as we eat only muscle meat which does not have this hormonal and protomorphic component.

He believed them to be highly implicated in auto-immune disease (AID) which he understood to be a *failure of repair* not a true disease in the sense of an acute disease model of one cause/one symptom. Instead it is the body's release of the PMs as the tissue becomes degraded and necrotic, with the resultant broken down tissue protein leaching out into the bloodstream, which then sets up an immune response to that protein (antigen). The

---

[i] Often this is due to heavy metal toxicity – the thyroid attracts these and chlorine naturally

immune response is then triggered to recognise its own tissue as *foreign* and starts attacking the part of the body this tissue originated in. Hence the autoimmune cascade is "the body's attempt to preserve itself, even though its effects could be more deadly than the disease itself". This would be true of all AID including heart disease, Hashimoto's thyroiditis, arthritis and so on. The solution as far as Dr Lee was concerned was to administer these nucleoproteins orally and their presence in the gut then *acts as a decoy* to the immune system to stop destroying the originating tissue. According to Tom Cameron, "their job is to help maintain normal cell metabolism and cell cycling, and to potentially enable tissue-specific immune downregulation."

It is an intriguing idea which has shown considerable success in animals[43]. If you are struggling to believe this could be a scientifically validated understanding, then consider the similarities to the concept of 'oral tolerance' which *is* accepted by the mainstream. Here an antigenic protein is administered orally to help induce tolerance by activating the T-Regulatory cells (which help balance immune response) and 'reboot' the immune system so it stops reacting to the antigen in a dose-dependent manner. Eventually the body stops reacting to the antigen altogether (**anergy**)[i]. This is accepted science but protomorphology is not. It's just bad timing for Dr Lee I think that his theories were overshadowed by Watson and Crick's DNA structure. Do look into it if you can – vets use it so why not doctors?

Environmental Threats and Toxicity

Glyphosate and the ECM

Research by Stephanie Seneff, senior research scientist at the Massachusetts Institute of Technology (MIT) in the US, has shown us that the negative ionic nature of structural glycoproteins (GAGs) means they attract positively charged molecules like heavy metals, and in particular the sulphate tails of the molecule attract **glyphosate**, the common herbicide applied routinely to our crops as Roundup[44].

Now, glyphosate is known for its toxicity – I wrote about this extensively in my previous book 'The World Within' but suffice to say glyphosate is a 'probable carcinogen'[ii], neurotoxin, and may well be implicated in

---

[i] This happens too by taking local honey regularly which successfully cured me of hayfever.
[ii] As defined by the World Health Organisation or WHO

gastrointestinal dysregulation by encouraging leaky gut. 'Roundup' (the formulation most used commercially) is even more toxic than the glyphosate itself as it contains surfactants and other toxic chemicals which make it even more potent as a herbicide. After decades of use, it has become ubiquitous in the soil and water. So it's almost impossible to avoid even if you eat all organic foods.[i] This is because it is routinely sprayed on crops to dessicate them prior to harvest, and that spray drifts in the air and then drains to the water system, even if you never eat a conventionally grown crop in your life, you can't escape it. Worse still, **GMO (genetically modified organism)** foods have been bred to withstand *even larger doses* than regular crops, so the intake when you eat those is huge. As a **chelator** (binder) of minerals[ii], it also promotes uptake of heavy metals from the gut into the brain and other tissues causing a huge rise in neurodegenerative disease as we will see in the Chapter 7.

Glyphosate is an amino acid (protein building block) very similar in structure to the amino acid glycine in the ECM which it largely displaces[45].

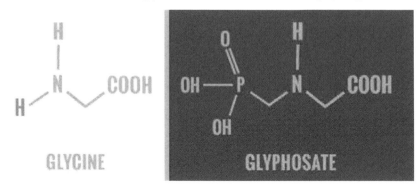

Figure 30: Glycine and Glyphosate Similarity

When this happens chaos ensues – proteins are informational molecules, the basis of life in the body. The information is largely transmitted by the protein's 3-D shape or conformation in space and this depends on the

---

[i] It might be strongly linked to coeliac disease with which it shares a common etiology.
[ii] It is by binding minerals and making them unusable to plants that it acts as a herbicide. It used to be thought of as safe because it doesn't do that to human cells. However, that was before we discovered what it does to the microbiome. GMO plants are designed with a small segment of a gene which is resistant to the glyphosate so they can be sprayed and survive but the weeds do not.

sequence of amino acids (basic building blocks) in the chain. If you change one amino acid in the chain, the shape of the molecule in space changes.

Glycine is a very simple amino acid with just a few atoms in the molecule – see above. When the hydrogen atom normally attached to the nitrogen atom in glycine has been replaced by a much bulkier and negatively-charged phosphorous-containing side chain in glyphosate, this stops the protein folding properly and binding its substrate (the thing that attaches to it in enzyme reactions). This small substitution has a massive effect therefore.

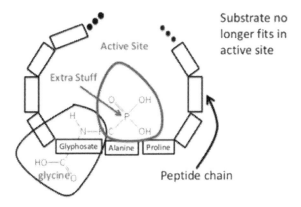

Figure 31: Glyphosate and Protein Structure

Most recently it has been implicated in gut issues seen with autism and IBS where gut motility is affected. According to Stephanie Seneff, the smooth muscle cells of our gut lining (responsible for gut motility) have glycine in the myosin protein. Myosin is the contractile protein that provides the contractions that propel food along the gut[i]. If the glycine[ii] is substituted by alanine (another amino acid) gut motility is reduced by 99%! Imagine then what happens when glyphosate replaces it.

But the gall bladder also uses muscle contraction to squirt out bile into the gut when digesting a fatty meal. So bile release is affected which may account for poor digestion of fats in some people (me included[iii]). Glyphosate also prevents bile production in the liver by interference with

[i] The same protein also creates muscular contraction in skeletal muscles but not smooth
[ii] at position 699 in the protein amino acid chain for all you geeks out there
[iii] Unfortunately in my previous career as a garden designer and plantswoman I was exposed to large amounts of glyphosate unwittingly as I thought it was safe to use.

CYP enzymes which are responsible for its manufacture. It affects the digestive enzymes, particularly trypsin, pepsin (both protein digesting enzymes) and lipase (for fat digestion). This typically causes pale stools with undigested particles and of course "**cholestasis** (stagnant bile) and the build-up of gall stones, eventually requiring the gall bladder to be removed[46]" . Gall bladder removal without dealing with the root cause is another travesty of modern medicine which ignores the imbalance, choosing instead to remove the 'warning light'.

There are other effects of glyphosate on our gut lining. As I said in my previous book The World Within:

"It destroys the gaps between lining cells (so called 'tight junctions') which control what molecules come in and out of our bloodstream). Glyphosate destroys our health over the long term therefore, so its use is tantamount to chemical poisoning of the food we eat (another reason to go organic in your diet!) and to add specific foods with high inulin (prebiotic) content that help to heal it. ... Fifty years of chemical agriculture has denuded the soil to a huge extent. A concentration of high doses of just three minerals (nitrogen, phosphorus and potassium - NPK fertiliser) has unbalanced the soil and the routine dosing with herbicides, pesticides and other chemical additives has killed off the valuable soil microorganisms (bacteria and fungi) that help to maintain a balance in the same way as in our bodies. Hence there are fewer insects to feed on the worms and then less wildlife that can live off the insects. It is frightening how much mineral and vitamins our vegetables have lost in 60 years of industrial agriculture.[47] What we do eat is lacking the essential nutrients they once obtained from the soil. No wonder we are all deficient and yet overfed!"[48]

If you doubt that glyphosate is anything other than safe (as I did), then just consider for a minute how it works to kill weeds. According to Seneff again:

"Such a substitution (glyphosate for glycine) within the protein EPSP synthase is by far the most plausible explanation for how it disrupts this critical enzyme in the Shikimate (energy producing) pathway in plants. Disruption of this enzyme is acknowledged by Monsanto as being the most damaging effect that it has on weeds"[49]

Why would this be accepted but not acknowledged in humans? I leave you to ponder. We revisit glyphosate again in Chapter 7 as it is crucial.

GMO's and Gut Bacterial Modification

In the last 40 or 50 years we have developed many new hybrids by crossing one species with another to improve food production. But with scientific advances in DNA modification technologies, we can now introduce genes from one species directly ('splicing') to give the recipient species characteristics from the donor. Hence, we can introduce genes that make a crop resistant to disease, for instance. But we do this by adding genes from bacteria and viruses that were never designed to be in plants – ones that decimate our internal bacterial population when we eat them. This is the essential problem with GMO foods – they interact with our microbiome in ways which are unpredictable and they swap genes between plants too via cross-pollination. So, non GMO crops which are in adjacent fields may also be affected. It is surely the greatest threat to our health aside from general chemical toxicity,

Toxicity - Persistent Organic Pollutants and Heavy Metals

We are subject to an unprecedented number of toxins in the environment, whether in the air we breathe, the clothes we wear, the water we drink or the food we eat. Never before in the history of life on this planet, have there been so many new chemicals introduced, previously unknown to life. This causes a potential problem as there are few microbes that have evolved which can digest or deactivate these chemicals. Of course, that is changing through mutation and natural selection, but it is a slower process than the rate at which we are releasing new products into the environment.

Persistent Organic Pollutants (POPs) are everywhere. Plasticisers like Bisphenol A (BPA), a common component of flexible plastic (as in plastic bottles), actually disrupts our body chemistry directly to form cancer cells. And BPB which has been produced to replace it is no better in fact may be worse. They are what are called a **xeno-oestrogens** and distort the body's hormonal function.

Other chemicals to watch out for are dioxins, phthalates (in personal care products), fire retardants, organophosphates, and glyphosate. Fat tissue is a dumping ground for many of these chemicals, as is the thyroid which is designed to concentrate iodine which is easily displaced by POP's; it's one of the hidden causes of the rise in breast cancer and thyroid issues that no-one talks about.

It is safer to decant the food into glass, stainless steel or enamel containers (depending on whether you're using conventional or microwave ovens, of course). Avoid non-stick pans, particularly if they are old and scratched/damaged. The heavy metal content seems to accumulate in the food and therefore you will ingest it gradually. Use iron frying pans as the iron they leach is actually helpful, particularly for women with thyroid issues who are often anaemic.

"Most people (even new born babies) have a considerable amount of chemical toxicity. A typical list of contaminants would be: DDT, PCBs, trichloroethylene, perchlorate, dibenzofurans, mercury, lead, benzene and arsenic. .. One of the worst places for chemicals is the home: plug in room deodorisers, perfumes, flame-retardants (on our sofas and carpets), dry-cleaning fluids, toilet deodorisers, cosmetic additives, cleaning products, gasoline by-products (Vaseline for instance), home pesticides and decorating products like paint thinners and wood preservatives. ... We have largely replaced natural cleaning products for nice-smelling chemical substitutes that make us feel good about ourselves in having a 'clean' (read sterile) home[50]"

Mercury is increasingly found in fish, like tuna, that are higher up the food chain. It is the second most poisonous chemical known to man – especially when it combines with organic chemicals in the body to form methyl mercury compounds e.g. from amalgam. Lead is found at chronic low levels in old houses too from lead paint.

Medications

Antibiotics have direct effects on our health too, mostly related to killing off our natural microbiome. But some have more direct effects: the antibiotic, tetracycline, for example, can block mineral absorption by binding with minerals, such as calcium, magnesium, iron and zinc in the GI tract. Nutrients are essential to the metabolic activities of every cell in the body. Some drugs deplete nutrients by speeding up the metabolic rate (hence their use in fattening up animals for slaughter). These drugs include antibiotics (including penicillin and gentamicin), steroids such as prednisone, and gout medication such as colchicine. Other drugs block nutrient production at the cellular level:

"medications can influence enzymes or receptors that help process essential nutrients. For example, widely prescribed statin drugs block the activity of Hydroxy-methyl-glutaryl coenzyme Q10 (HMG-CoA), an enzyme that's required to manufacture cholesterol in the body. This action also depletes the body of the important protein molecule coenzyme Q10 (CoQ10), which requires HMG-CoA for its production. This has a serious negative impact on muscle and heart health. Anyone taking statins should also take CoQ10 as a supplement. In some countries this is now routinely recommended though not, sadly, in the UK.[51] Drugs also can increase the loss of nutrients through the urinary system. Any drug that does this can drain the body's levels of water-soluble nutrients, including B vitamins and minerals, such as magnesium and potassium. The major offenders are medications to treat hypertension, particularly the diuretics that reduce blood pressure by increasing the volume of water flushed out of the body."[i]

Heavy Metal Toxicity

Some people are especially susceptible to environmental toxins due to their particular genetic predisposition and their type of exposure. Metals differ in their toxicity – particularly damaging are positively charged metal ions (like aluminium and mercury) which bind to negatively charged molecules (ions) found naturally in the human system. These organic ions combine to make a new compound with the heavy metal which makes them even more damaging e.g. methyl mercury, 'a highly toxic form that builds up in fish, shellfish and animals that eat fish. Fish and shellfish are the main sources of methyl-mercury exposure to humans'.[52] Although dental amalgam ('silver') fillings are also a low but consistent source in the body – they are in fact 55% mercury the second most potent neurotoxin known to man.

Inside the Home

This is an area that is seldom considered. If you asked most people where the worst source of toxicity was, they would probably talk about the external environment of diesel particulates, PCB's, heavy metals, etc. But it's a little known fact that your home environment can be more toxic than your outside environment. A recent study showed that air quality inside many homes (especially new ones with the off-gassing of new furniture and carpets) is very low. Old houses may have damp and therefore be releasing silent invisible mould spores into the air. And because most people have double glazed, sealed homes, there is little air movement so toxic gases can build up to dangerous levels.

---

[i] If you or anyone you know is on these medications, you must take mineral supplements away from your medication to replenish the stores. Cramp is a cardinal sign of depletion.

Mould

With older homes with poor insulation, condensation can be a real issue which encourages the growth of mould (fungus). In addition if that home has had water-damage and there's mould growth in the building itself (sometimes an old problem of which the current inhabitants are unaware) *and* if a person is intolerant of mould[i], health problems will undoubtedly ensue. This is because mould produces silent, microscopic, invisible **mycotoxins** in the spores (a form of systemic biotoxin), arguably more toxic than heavy metals. They affect vision, in particular visual acuity, as they impair oxygen capacity in the optic nerve; this is used as a functional test of likely infestation[ii].

But other more obvious symptoms include brain fog and forgetting words, red eyes, joint pain, static electricity shocks (yes really – due to excess chloride on the skin from poor hydration regulation as mould affects the pituitary)[53], poor blood sugar control (as it interferes with pancreatic function) and weight gain (due to the dysregulation of satiety peptide leptin-adiponectin function). It often ties in with other conditions like Lyme Disease (an overgrowth of a group of bacteria including Borelia, Bartinella and other microbes[iii]), which arguably are the body's attempt to rid itself of the toxin rather than the 'disease' itself.

There are other deep effects at a cellular level too. For instance, in the presence of biotoxic mould, your glutathione (the body's most powerful detox system) will have been exhausted from continual detoxification of the biotoxins and **volatile organic chemicals (VOC's)** that mould produces. It is hard to know whether mould is a problem for you unless you test for it with a nutritional therapist or functional medicine doctor. But if you are suffering persistent chronic symptoms despite having improved your diet and lifestyle and your answer yes to any of the questions below, then suspect mould.

---

[i] A particular Human Leukocyte Antigen HLA-DR gene SNP which changes the antigen presentation system within the immune system – approx. 24% of the population.
[ii] A good test for biotoxic illness is a vision test called the Visual Contrast Sensitivity Test VCS test available on vcstest.com and survivingmold.com for a small fee.
[iii] According to expert Dr Dietrich Klinghardt, Lyme is not the same in the US and Europe – the US version has altered viral particles associated with the many pathogenic bacteria which would explain both its virulence and difficulties in applying one cure for all.

Biotoxic exposure Quiz

1. Do musty odours bother you?
2. Have you worked or lived in a building where the air vents were discoloured or where there is water damage or discoloration on ceilings or elsewhere?
3. Has your home ever been flooded or had leaks in the roof?
4. Do you experience shortness of breath/ recurring sinus infections/ recurring bronchial infections and coughing/flu-like symptoms?
5. Do you notice an increase of symptoms on rainy days?
6. Do you have frequent headaches?
7. Are you fatigued and have a skin rash?

The symptoms you will experience depend on what you have been exposed to, for how long and how your body responds to that exposure (which of course is individual). First you have to check what exposures you've had and there are a variety of tests that can be run to check this (shown in the table overleaf).

Table 1: Markers of Mould Exposure

VCS	positive	Visual Contrast Sensitivity Test – do this first then if positive see a practitioner for the following tests
HLA-DR	positive	Human Leucocyte Antigen. Immune marker of auto-immunity
VEF-F	High Normal 31-86 pg/mL	Vascular endothelial growth factor (VEGF) high initially shows extra capillary growth to help protect the blood delivery of oxygen
TGF-β1	<2380 pg/ml	a master regulator of the immune system above even T-Regs
MSH	<30 Normal 35-81 pg/mL	Melanocyte Stimulating Hormone – affects sleep and suppresses appetite, increases aromatase to cause oestrogen dominance, saltwater balance, adrenal/thyroid dys-reulation – likely hypothyroid[i].
MMP-9	high	Degrades the extracellular matrix (ECM)

---

[i] Adding extra thyroid hormone does not help these people and they may have been diagnosed as simply hypothyroid when really they have mould exposure. See Dr Jill Carnahan

The extracellular matrix (ECM) will be systematically degraded by enzymes called **matrix metalloproteins (MMP)**, with the result that the MMP-9 level will be elevated[i]. This is a form of matrix dysregulation which can be exacerbated by taking quinolone antibiotics, which act by degrading matrix proteins further. MMP-9 is one of the markers of mould exposure.

The environmental remedy can be expensive if you need your cavity walls cleaned out or you have to move! However, there are simple things you can do to alleviate (though not eradicate) this problem:

1. Use a diffuser with frankincense and citrus oils. Frankincense in particular is very powerfully anti-fungal in this respect.
2. Make sure you ventilate your home properly – even when cold. Open windows for 10-20 mins in the morning to allow fresh air in.
3. If condensation is an obvious problem then get a dehumidifier too – and especially if you dry washing on radiators indoors.
4. Install a HEPA air filter. Make sure it is ion free (a source of ozone)
5. Take glutathione, vitamin C, NAC, ALA (and possibly binders like Cholestyramine under the supervision of a qualified practitioner).[ii]
6. Reduce EMF exposure by turning off WiFi at night and/or shielding yourself with a laptop guard like Harapad or wearing biodots. If using a cellphone never hold it to your head but use earbuds or put it on speaker phone. Use a corded landline if possible or put on speaker phone rather than close to head. Put it on airplane mode (offline) while you sleep. Never have your router in your bedroom.

Don't assume that a new home is immune from these problems; new houses can have very poor ventilation. And the higher your Wi-Fi exposure, the more mycotoxins your fungi produce so if you live in flats/condominiums or in close proximity to other's EMF's or with smart meters[iii] you can get sicker as your mould gets 'threatened'[54].

Toxins are everywhere and we still don't know the cumulative effect of low doses in combination. In a recent American study, babies were found to have 300 industrial pollutants in their cord blood! So, toxicity begins even before you are born, via the placental blood supply in the womb. You are born with these PCB, DDT, and even dioxins which have been banned for

---

[i] Amongst other see table 1. As not everyone has this it needs to be on combination with other markers. As not everyone is sensitive these people may not be believed and be accused of making it up.

[ii] See list by Dr Ritchie Shumaker on survivingmold.com.

[iii] Smart meters are huge emitters of EMR and so their installation should be shielded if you are sensitive.

30 years! The reason they're still there, even though we no longer use them, is they don't break down. Some are particularly bad as they are fat soluble and endocrine (hormone) disruptors. In the endocrine system, low doses can have a huge effect[i] . Refer to The World Within for more info.

---

[i] See the 'dirty dozen' on the EWG.com website

Chapter 4: The Brain, Stress and Environment

The Brain

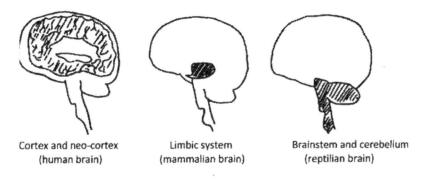

| Cortex and neo-cortex | Limbic system | Brainstem and cerebellum |
| (human brain) | (mammalian brain) | (reptilian brain) |

Figure 32: Three Evolutionary Stages of the Human Brain

The brain is not just a lump of fatty tissue; it is complex and hierarchical. It developed in 3 layers often referred to as the Triune Brain Model. This diagram shows us those 3 layers in diagrammatic form. Note that these three layers basically go from the outside layer (cortex) of the conscious brain to the deeper bottom layer (brainstem). It's like a series of brains wrapped one on top of the other. Although this model has been altered over the years, it is still one that helps in explaining some of the functions of the brain that are *unconscious* as the majority of brain function is. Not only do these three layers correspond to evolutionary development of the human from more primitive animals it also corresponds **phylogenetically** i.e. the development of the human from conception onwards.

Brain Development

When we are first born our brains are immature; our pre-frontal cortex (PFC – the planning centre) is offline. We are born with the older, more primitive parts of our brain intact – the brainstem and limbic system. This is enough to control certain innate behaviours such as suckling (via brainstem), but then our limbic system begins to develop to allow us to orient to safety and develop emotional regulation and bonding skills. This is a crucial time for brain formation as the brain is growing at an astonishing rate. Around the age of seven the cortex begins to mature and the child can begin to make analysis of its environment (a sort of rudimentary 'risk/benefit analysis'!). The child is then able to delay gratification for longer term benefit[i].

Sex differentiation begins with conception – with the foetal sex hormones coming online in the first trimester. The release of testosterone from the instruction of XY chromosome makes a male brain[ii]. This has profound implications throughout life; with more testosterone, for instance, the male brain is encouraged in certain pursuit behaviours e.g. aggression. Girls have fifteen times the level of oestrogen compared to boys with the result they are driven to need to be attractive (whereas boys are more concerned with pursuit). It's official – their brains are different! [iii] There is much that can go awry, for instance if some genetic mutations occur, the androgen receptor is non-functioning and the body will become more female. We see this with some boys/men who develop breasts for instance. But this may be a toxicity issues interacting with the genes[iv].

There are profound differences between the sexes, for instance, in the 0-3 month phase: eye gaze in the baby girl will increase by 400% in that time - which doesn't occur in little boys. So, in other words, girls watch moving objects around them better, presumably as a bonding mechanism (women tend towards the 'tend and befriend' (parasympathetic) pattern neurologically rather than 'fight and flight' (sympathetic system). I know we

---

[i] Recent studies have shown that children who are able to do this perform better in life.
[ii] The default is female, so if nothing intervenes, the foetus would always be female.
[iii] That's not to say that environment doesn't have a big part to play, but the 'gun' is loaded in this direction, for the environment to then pull the trigger. Please note I am not talking about *gender* differences, which is a social (environmental) construct.
[iv] Many persistent organic pollutants in water act as xeno-estrogens and can feminise

would rather believe that baby's brains are blank slates but as any parent will tell you, their baby girls and boys have innate differences.

There is then a second spurt around puberty when hormones start to increase again. For instance, if there is overgrowth of the adrenals 'adrenal hyperplasia' then girls may make more testosterone from their adrenals and become same-sex attracted. Presumably a failure of testosterone production in boy children at that age may affect their sexuality too, perhaps becoming more feminised, and possibly gay. Certainly the teenage brain is 'under construction' and many things can affect it, for good or ill. Of course the parenting environment influences this too and our gender culture (which people in the transgender movement now term 'binary') is much more influential in the later years of childhood.

In girls, puberty begins the ovarian production of oestradiol, one of the oestrogens that controls the female cycle. It is highest around ovulation (as is testosterone for sex drive – all in order to ensure fertilisation of the egg). In the latter half of the cycle progesterone increases (which makes you feel good until it suddenly drops triggering pre-menstrual syndrome (PMS), irritability and an 'out of sorts' feeling) and then finally menstruation and release (phew!). Most people are familiar with the female cycle in terms of hormones but are perhaps less clear on how this affects the brain – I include here an image that pulls this together showing how and why women have neurological changes (in mood, drive, etc) over their cycle.

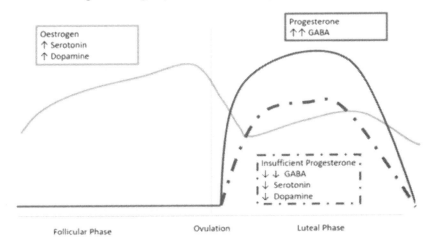

Figure 33: Female Neuroendocrine Cycle

85

Note that the idealised variation (in green and blue solid lines[i]) is co-ordinated so progesterone goes up[ii] when oestrogen goes down. Much can go wrong though, when progesterone (which needs cholesterol for its manufacture) is in short supply, levels of happy neurotransmitters GABA serotonin and dopamine can go down. Then a woman can feel very much less energetic, connected and vital. It is particularly sad that young women and teenage girls, who should be in the prime of life, suffer the debilitating symptoms of depression and energy drain given this scenario, brought on by stress and low fat diets. One of the worst effects of social media is to hook in to girl's sense of needing approval and magnify it. So that instead of your small social circle, who you generally know, you are forced to compete with hundreds of people you barely interact with outside of the online medium. For young women, biologically wired as they are to compete with one another for the attraction of a mate, it can be devastating and the rise in social media use may be a significant factor in teenage mental ill health particularly amongst girls and young women[55,56].

Stress and Emotional Health

Stress is an enormous factor in health and wellbeing. It is not a vague concept as understood colloquially, but a *physiological mechanism*, which sets in motion a cascade of changes in the body, which are collectively called '**the stress response**'. In my first book, I looked in detail at the stress response and how it relates to physical and mental health[11]. I won't repeat the detail here but there are some important principles to understand with regard to the concept of stress that many people misunderstand. Stress is a natural fact of life, but its nature is very variable; it is not just the overt stress that we *perceive* that causes problems. There can be different types of stress (including positive stress or **eustress**), but it is the *unconscious unrelenting* kind (**toxic stress**) that causes the most problems for people with regard to their physical and mental health as they don't always perceive it is happening.

So, firstly what is stress? Physiologically, stress is anything that takes the body out of **homeostasis** i.e. toxins, trauma[iii], and negative beliefs which perpetuate an inflammatory neuro-hormonal cascade of cytokines,

---

i This wonderful diagram was drawn by my colleague Emma Chapman-Sharp
ii In pregnancy it gradually increases over the nine months
iiiTrauma is sdefined as anything that overwhelms our capacity to cope .e.g. abuse, surgery, abandonment, bereavement, etc to an unsupported/sensitised person (esp. children).

prostaglandins and so on (I go into more detail on this cellular response in the later chapters on disease states). As I have intimated already, stress can become *a learned response to threat*, particularly if this was the default state when you were growing up. It can therefore become chronic if not relieved in adulthood, as the brain adapts by developing a lower threshold to stress – something that is termed '**kindling**'. This is because the wiring of the brain is such that the more certain nerve pathways are followed, the easier it becomes to follow them in future – it's as if the road becomes wider the more it is travelled! This then becomes your default response to certain triggers, such that it may develop into 'a habit of being', which makes anxiety and depression much more likely.

So, far from being irrelevant or too long ago to matter, "early emotional trauma such as an unloving mother, accidents, bullying, or ill health landscape the brain for more trauma later in life. This traumatic memory is stored in the unconscious parts of the brain as a survival response which is easily retriggered and can cause myriad seemingly unexplained medical symptoms throughout the body. The most common, though, are chronic pain, digestive issues and skin complaints."[49]

Brain Neuroplasticity in Health and Disease

How does the brain store these messages of threat or pain? Well there is a strange ability of the brain to adapt and grow its neuronal connections (**neuroplasticity**), dependent on the environment, particularly in early childhood. If the parents are supportive, the brain develops normally with good connections, stress is mitigated by self-soothing behaviours which enhances *resilience* - the ability of that child to withstand stress. Without good attunement with the parents, children develop a low stress tolerance and hyper-reactivity.

Moreover, neuroplasticity is not limited to childhood; in fact, recent imaging studies of the brain have given us a very clear idea that the brain, particularly areas like the hippocampus, are able to change dynamically *throughout its lifetime*. This is both good news and bad news. If the environment is good then we can adapt to produce good connections across different brain regions. If our environment is poor, then the changes will enhance survival (but not 'thrival'[i]) by downplaying creativity, joy and

---

[i] I've invented this word but it explains that the body will prioritise basic survival even at the expense of quality of life.

connection. One of the most important environmental signals for resilience is our relationships with others – particularly those with whom we have an emotional bond.

The Interpersonal Neurobiology of Relationships

We are social beings; wired to connect with each other. We connect with others throughout our life experience – from birth to death. But the early life experience is the most crucial as the brain is immature at birth and largely shaped and moulded by experience (due to the neuroplasticity (re-wire-ability) of the brain.

Attachment Theory and Poor Attunement

Attachment is the term given to the bonds you make with your caregivers early in life, and it is a very crucial interplay of stimulus and response. In a **secure attachment** (approximately 30% of the population) the mother (and later on father) and baby mutually regulate each other and the parent can anticipate the needs of the child such that it feels secure in its 'I-ness'. However if a child's needs aren't met consistently for whatever reason, then an **insecure attachment** forms which can be characterised as anxious (clingy /ambivalent) or avoidant (dissociative, seemingly calm but actually distressed) personalities. Finally, if needs aren't reliably met at all then a disorganised attachment pattern is adopted, life become chaotic and certain symptoms emerge. The problem with these childhood patterns (actually formed very early on), is that they are *unconscious* and become **conditioned** i.e. habitual. People then carry these patterns on into their adolescence and adulthood where they wreak havoc with relationships with peers and partners.

(30%) – needs are met consistently.
Able to self-soothe. Mother and child are *mutually regulated** – they understand each other instinctively and are able to regulate each other automatically

Insecure: ambivalent/anxious – child is both drawn to and repelled by caregiver – preference for auto-(other) regulation but not by mother. Child seeks contact but then pulls away. Confused and confusing. Become *anxious adults* (focussed on past failure) High cortisol

Insecure: avoidant – will reject parent and show preference for distraction (self-regulation) rather than connection. Become *dismissive adults*, unable to emote. Low cortisol

Disorganised – nothing works! Highly dysregulated autonomically** – show dissociative tendencies (fainting, trancelike states, rocking, bed-wetting, addictive/compulsive behaviours)

Figure 34: Attachment Strategies

The successful making and survival of relationships is not just about psychology, it has a chemical basis in the brain. For instance, lust comes from a surge of the hormone testosterone[i], falling in love gives the brain a huge rush of dopamine (the 'seeking' neurotransmitter) and **noradrenaline** (drive or motivation). After a while, as reality bites and your rose-tinted view of the other begins to seem less accurate as differences emerge, the levels decrease and then other brain chemicals take over, primarily **oxytocin** (the bonding hormone). This is the beginning of intimacy, which requires the tolerance of differences, and the ability to tolerate closeness (read by the body as immobilisation) *without fear*.

Believe it or not, this is a really big problem for many people (including myself it turns out). If you have had any trauma in your history, your brain will interpret intimacy as a *threat*, and instinctively recoil. This is because the mammalian brain is wired to learn from past experience, and it maps out its memories of the appropriate responses within the limbic system as implicit (wordless) memories. If, in your childhood, the relationship with your parent was less than reliable, it is termed insecure, and your tendency with

---

[i] Men having generally higher levels might account for the higher sex drive of men and the greater nurturance need of women.

others will be to feel threatened by intimate love relationships. Indeed Dr Dan Brown, co-author of The Attachment Project, states that complex (relational) trauma is really untreated insecure or disorganized attachment![57]

Happy love relationships have high health benefits, as the bonding hormone oxytocin (brought about by physical touch mainly) directly lowers the stress hormone cortisol. But conversely, *poor* relationships cause chronic stress and high cortisol, which promotes premature ageing by epigenetic means (shortened telomeres on DNA, poor cellular energy production, etc). So stress is inflammatory in more ways than one!

Happy couples may still fight, but they are not as **autonomically** dysregulated[i], there is still enough respect for the other and a tolerance of vulnerability, that compromise is possible. Physically there will still be plenty of eye contact and body contact is resumed when making up. This requires a certain amount of emotional intelligence, a willingness to tolerate differences and trust of oneself and the other. Eye contact is absolutely necessary, as it helps regulate the emotions of the other, as is a certain perception of the other as 'special' and therefore worth spending time over[ii]. Happy couples mend easily as they trust they can repair the hurt and disconnect of a breach of relationship. In many ways relationships are a balance of self-protection and attachment. Unfortunately in today's society, the trend has been to 'look out for number one' rather than each other, so it is not culturally validated to compromise or work on differences. Hence the high divorce rate one could argue.

Arguments and disagreements, whilst natural in all relationships, can be particularly devastating for those whose early life attunement was insecure. When you are criticised for instance, your brain automatically registers danger – the **amygdala** in your emotional brain (**limbic system**) is triggered in the here and now, but also by old emotional memories that are re-awakened. Both the unconscious parts of your brain become awash in cortisol (the main stress hormone) and therefore highly dysregulated and reactive. There may be a knee-jerk reaction to defensiveness (mediated by the fight and flight hormonal cascade of the HPA axis). It may result in an

---

[i] The autonomic nervous system is responsible for our most basic automatic functions of breathing, heart rate and digestion. But it shares links with the social bonding system and relaying of expressions via eyes, voice and body language.
[ii] And I would argue a sense of self-worth is vital too as seeing yourself as important, valuable and worthy of love is intrinsic to perceiving love.

unstoppable impulse to blame the other. We justify our reactions by rationalising our reactivity without realising we are in 'Fear Central' and both participants are doing the 'dance of the amygdalas' as neuroscientist Joseph LeDoux has wittily called it[58].

In addition, as your brain is biased towards the negative (it notices negative things more easily than positive, and thoughts generally are about 85% negative), we find fault in our partner (or ourselves) or find ourselves going down the road of focussing on what wrong rather than what's right. Love and trust needs to be nurtured, i.e. worked upon. How then do we avoid falling into the trap our emotional brains have unwittingly set for us? This is the job of the **pre-frontal cortex (PFC)** and one could view it as the balance to the amygdala's job of unthinking reactivity to old emotional memories.

The amygdala is online at birth and one of its tasks is to mark those events which have emotional significance, particularly biased to the negative ones (the negativity bias is approximately 5:1). However, it's not all bad; it is needed for empathy and the assessment of trust. But it needs to be regulated properly by the balancing pre-frontal cortex (PFC) – part of the thinking brain.

The Prefrontal Cortex and Resilience

The PFC comes online gradually from ages 6/7 through to your mid-20's (a little later for men) but a lesser known fact is that it continues to change throughout the lifespan. It is intrinsic to social behavior and morality (along with deeper brain regions like the **anterior cingulate cortex** (ACC)[i] and **hippocampus**) . It has myriad links both across left and right hemispheres (horizontally) and vertically which help it to access contextual information, such as 'what is the meaning of this', 'when did this last happen?' or 'do I need to be afraid'. There are some genetic differences between people as to how well this operates, but it is mostly an environmental influence that wires us well or dysfunctionally.

According to trauma therapist, Janina Fisher, "when the PFC shuts down, we lose the part of the brain that witnesses our experience." The nearby hippocampus shrinks and instead of memory storage here as with normal

---

[i] Sometimes also called the cingulate gyrus in some textbooks

91

'explicit' memories, our raw, *unprocessed* memories become stored as sensory fragments within the limbic system (amygdala, etc). These 'implicit' memories have no words to describe them and because they are not available to conscious awareness (having lost the link to the cortex) may not be recognised as the memories they are.

The first most people know of them is the bodily symptoms they evoke: pain, tingling, numbness, stiffness, etc. Triggers of these emotional memories can be very subtle: from the time of day, shifts in body language of another, emotions that are unacceptable (e.g. rage), smells, separation/loss, and so on. Because many of the originating experiences were had before our cortex came online, we have no context (including awareness of it being in the past) with which to counter them. We may have shattering dreams or nightmares, but no idea what they are about. And the more triggers we have, the more easily the response is evoked (so-called kindling). We are in neural disarray.

Experiences vary, but most people avoid or fight their internal sensations to the point of becoming phobic of them, and the downward cycle into illness is assured as the cellular effects of toxic stress messages continues unabated day after day. If we want to have health, happy relationships, we have to strengthen our resilience to stress.

Managing Chronic Stress

We need to both recognise and then manage the broad array of stresses that we are under. It is not as simple as avoiding stressful situations. Firstly, many of them will be *unconscious*, and secondly some of them will be unavoidable. But, given that every life will have stresses of one sort or another, and most childhoods have some trauma, how do we actually achieve this?

The Brain and Resilience

Given that our PFC could be considered the regulator of our emotional reactivity, we could consider it the 'CEO of resilience', as Linda Graham has called it. How to we engage the PFC without becoming dysregulated? The answer, in one word is safety. Or should I be more precise? It is the stimulus of feeling safe *in one's body* which enables the PFC to come online and dampen the amygdalae[i] and other danger response centres[ii]. Now, I am emphasizing the somatic (body) component because I am not talking about physical safety in the world. We can't really control that, after all. This is more to do with how you feel in the world; whether you feel you have a place, a purpose and a means to develop that purpose (agency/meaning). Many children grow up never feeling safe in their home environment for various reasons and this landscapes their brain to expect unsafety and scan for it – this is the basis of **hypervigilance**. So, safety has to be (re-)learned if this is the case. Thankfully due to the adult brain's remaining plasticity, this is possible with the right techniques.

Stephen Porges, author of ground-breaking **polyvagal theory**, emphasises what he calls '**neuroception**' as the gateway to this internal sense. Neuroception is the awareness of your internal body state as safe or not (whether tense, relaxed, etc) and it is no exaggeration to say that some of my clients have *no bodily sense of themselves at all*, let alone a safe one. This is a sad state of affairs that comes about particularly where life stresses have been unremitting and support has been absent or insufficient; the brain effectively shuts down its experience of the body as being too painful. It is a highly dissociative state which may become normalised so the person hardly realises they are dissociating

In order to bring this back takes patience and practice. But firstly it is important to experience *vulnerability* whilst simultaneously being held in the mind and heart of another person (usually a therapist, or perhaps a good adult relationship). That positive experience and the resonant connection it engenders between the two people, enables the heart to open, oxytocin to flood the brain, and the PFC to come online as a compassionate observing presence; all pre-requisites for healing.

Once that is established, it is possible to come to terms with past experience as being *over* and choosing to do things differently in the present (i.e. not being dictated to by your habitual responses). Resilience, after all is the state of 'response flexibility' and this allows us to shift our awareness and come to acceptance of our reality, without fear. This is not the place to describe somatic-sensing therapies here, I refer the reader to the expert

---

i There are actually two amygdalae, one in the left brain and one in the right. They have slightly different functions but for simplicity can be thought of as the brain's smoke alarm.
ii I avoid calling it the 'fear centre' as Joseph LeDoux, who first studied the amygdala, claims his early work on this was misinterpreted and now prefers to call it the danger centre as fear is more likely the work of other higher brain areas which interpret the initial signal

texts on the matter[i] . But suffice to say, when safety is felt internally, change becomes not only possible but *inevitable.*

The importance of meaning

It was Frances Crick, one half of the duo who discovered DNA, who was purported to have written on his lab notice board 'meaning is everything'. Meaning would seem to be unique to humans with our higher mental functioning and evaluating brain. We are able to work out when something is 'right' for us – whether it offers us something that feels in keeping with a purpose deeper than mere existence (a spiritual awareness). When we ask people near the end of life what gave their life meaning, few answer their promotions, fancy cars or money. Most say things like their friends, their children, animals and for some it's the land they live on. In other words it is something with which they have a *relationship.* And that relationship is *felt inside the body* (particularly the heart) as of value. Few would argue that life has more purpose when it is full of meaning. But what is it about pursuing these meaningful relationships that affects your biology?

Living according to your values

I have long noticed that those who get ill are often those who have lost meaning in their lives in some way or other and are no longer living consistently with their values. I had no definitive explanation for this effect other than it was the interaction of the autonomic nervous system with the stress response. After all if you are living in a way that is not congruent with what you truly believe that is going to be a stress on the body. However, then I came across the work of Dr John Demartini. He eloquently describes the idea of 'telos' or the wisdom of the body which derives, in part from the homeostatic balance of our autonomic (sympathetic and parasympathetic nervous systems). These should be in homoeostatic balance over the day (as state of homeostasis or more correctly now termed allostasis).

When we perceive more support than challenge we will be in **parasympathetic dominance** (i.e. rest and digest). When we perceive more challenge than support we are more likely to exist in **sympathetic dominance** (fight and flight) – and if severe it will be perceived as trauma.

---

[i] The Scar that won't Heal by myself and 'Waking the Tiger' by Peter Levine

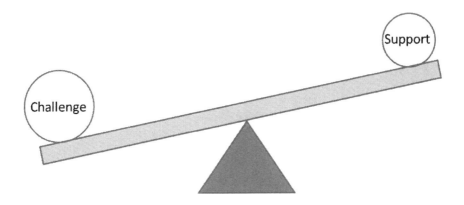

Sympathetic (fight and flight) = more challenge than support
(Parasympathetic (rest and digest) = more support than challenge)

Figure 35: Support vs. Challenge in Autonomic Nervous System
(adapted from Dr Martini)

Both these pathways have their own dominant hormones and neurotransmitters which influence the cell epigenetically. For instance in a parasympathetic repair state (a life lived according to our innate values) we will have a dominance of acetylcholine which interact with the cell membrane receptor to send a intra-cellular signal called cGMP which promotes genes for repair. The opposite is also true: when a life is lived with no reference to our innate values (or according to someone else's i.e. our parent's values) then the cellular message sent via cAMP interacts with the DNA to produce genes for breakdown.

Values are not generally looked at by most people unless they've done some psychotherapy which encourages it. At the Chrysalis Effect (a group I've trained with) their programme of CFS/ME recovery includes value determination exercises and encourages people to investigate their values and monitor how they are living according to them (or not). Perhaps that explains their phenomenal success rates with recovery. But if you are not on a programme like that and wish to investigate then there are many online resources that can help you discover yours. When you find that your life is not in alignment with them, it is a big impetus for change.

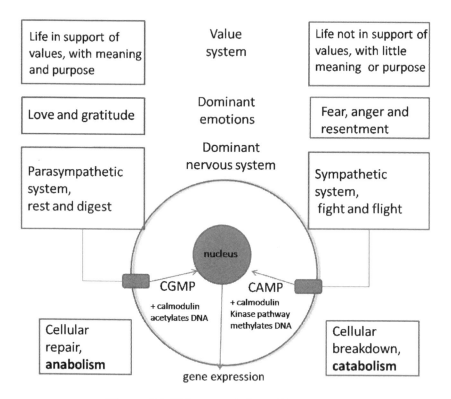

Figure 36: Values and Gene Expression
(adapted from Dr Martini)

So we see that values have a direct effect on whether defence and catabolism (breakdown) or growth and anabolism (construction) becomes more dominant. These cellular responses are also linked to which of your emotions i.e. love & gratitude versus resentment & anger are dominant. We have long known that those who live with anger, resentment or other negative emotions tend to have heart attacks or get other diseases more readily but now we have a mechanism for this epigenetic change. And because values are something we all have whether we are aware of them or not[i], we are able to investigate this and change our lives to suit. We can't always change our material circumstances, that is true but things like our relationships, self-worth, and focus are changeable with the right information. Making powerful choices to find love and harmony – even when a difficult situation is presenting itself is a skill which we can develop.

---

[i] We may have inherited some that we have never questioned from our parents or extended families but it important to find what our true values are live in accordance with them.

Values and meaning are highly linked. Because whatever is our highest value is what gives us meaning and purpose and it behoves us to find this and work with it to increase our 'flow' state. When we are in the flow, life becomes easier and we find more support than challenge (although we still need both). We find that even when bad things happen (which they will – expect them) we develop resilience; the ability to bounce back. How does one practically achieve this? Well we need to get present with the feelings and find the positive in it. To every situation there is a positive even if it isn't one we want. As an example if we fall ill – what could the positive be in that? Maybe it gives us the opportunity to rest with a chance to review our lives. Maybe we get more attention and sympathy which is missing. Values are driven by what we feel we lack and we seek more of. When you understand this you no longer blame yourself for beliefs and behaviours that seem illogical. So, when we find the hidden positive in the situation we shift our biology to a different state. This then becomes a cellular message of synthesis, synchronicity and a wholeness of being which is completely unconscious. It changes the balance of the cell towards repair and away from breakdown and thus extends both our longevity (via extending telomeres) and our wellness. So we are not only adding years to our life but life to our years!

But living according to our highest values or telos doesn't just change the cell but the brain too (with which the cells are connected via the neuroendocrine system). In particular, the **telencephalon** – (part of the forebrain including the pre-frontal cortex, and limbic structures of amygdala and hippocampus) is profoundly affected. The hippocampus in particular is one of the most plastic parts of the brain. It can grow new neurons over a few days and strengthen the existing connections in a few seconds – just from a thought or belief that are congruent with your true values.[i] How it does this is by the glial cells (the brain's immune cells) which helps to strengthen the nerve fibre by promoting myelination. Myelin is the protective sheath around the nerve fibre that acts like insulation around a wire. It makes the nerve fibres much, much faster. And this happens within milliseconds and is the basis for neuroplasticity (ability of the brain to remodel itself).

---

[i] These are not necessarily what you tell yourself your values are but your core values are identifiable from what you surround yourself with and what you devote most of your time to.

Many of us inherit our ideas of who we are from our parents and the kind of environment we grew up in. For some of us that environment wasn't ideal for some reason, e.g. a parent who was depressed, addicted or violent. For some it's just that we weren't 'right' for our parents in some way and so support was lacking. Trauma (unresolved emotional events) can be many things – it is an interpretation of the world that is basically frightening and unsupportive and it is stored unconsciously as a blueprint for how you are and 'how life is'.

So, the kinds of thoughts you think and your behaviours that are driven by your unquestioned belief system will create a story of your life that drives your biology. This may not be immediately apparent as it is an unconscious feedback system, but over a lifetime the effects of continual stress response of living in disharmony to our purpose (and each of us has an individual construction of that), will be felt in the body as disease. From this point of view, illness or symptoms are simply feedback and not to be feared, but responded to. Most people live in an internally constructed reality, not in the real world. We rely on the past (memory) and projections of the future (imagination) to guide us and this is interpreted bodily by our brains. Deepak Chopra believes it is what ages us; he calls it has called a "timeless mind and ageless body" When our mind is perfectly balanced it just has presence in the here and now and we feel inspired by our life and full of vitality. And our body symptoms, if we have any, dissolve – they are simply feedback that your life is out of balance in some way.

Learning to live a masterful life in balance with ones higher purpose allows us to move our focus from the imminent (human, material) to the transcendent (all-encompassing or divine) mind. If I haven't blown your mind yet, then there's no hope! I return to some of these more esoteric ideas in the last Chapter but for now, I leave you to ponder.

In the next chapter we delve into more detail how your biography translates into your biology of disease or wellness.

Chapter 5: Cellular Metabolism and Disease

Within a naturopathic understanding all diseases are manifestations of a different fault line i.e. a weak point but the *underlying problem is similar* so can be healed in similar ways. This is the exact opposite of modern medicine's approach that seeks to find the molecular pattern or organism that is different and *treat that*. This is particularly important understanding for neurodegenerative disorders that are thought by modern medicine to be disorders of the *brain*. Millions of pounds and dollars of government a research have gone towards understanding the minutiae of brain function as opposed to dealing with the underlying problem in the gut. We now know:

"the gut microbiome has a really important role to play in this; changes in the microbiome occur five years before diagnosis. This is largely a result of toxic build up in the brain (neurotoxicity). There are of course genetic predispositions; i.e. a genetic mutation can cause a build-up of particular metabolites in the brain for instance in **Parkinson's Disease** there is a genetic susceptibility in Dopamine metabolism[59].

It has been estimated that most disease is around 70% environmental and toxins have a huge part to play.

The old model that disease happens as the result of a one-time infection or assault (acute medicine) is no longer viable. We are seeing more and more **chronic disease** where the causative damage may have been a long time ago and it is the degradation of the *systems of repair* that initiate and keep the disease present. This is the new **functional/natural medicine** model which is slowly gaining ground. And the basis of this new model is the cell. According to Naviaux:

"all chronic diseases produce systems abnormalities that either block communication (signalling) or send alarm signals between cells and tissues. Cells that cannot communicate normally with neighboring or distant cells are

99

estranged from the whole, cannot reintegrate back into normal tissue and organ function and are functionally lost to the tissue. If the block in cell-cell communication occurs in a child, then the normal trajectory of development can be changed, leading to alterations in brain structure and function, and changes in long-term metabolic adaptations of other organs like liver, kidney, microbiome, and immune system. If the communication block occurs in adults, then organ performance is degraded over time, more and more cells with disabled or dysfunctional signalling accumulate, and age-related deterioration of organ function, senescence, or cancer occurs.[60].

Does this sound familiar to anyone – what is the disease that most represents this loss of control? I would venture cancer is that disease, the end-game as far as the body is concerned. But *there are always antecedents* – more modest diseases that pre-empt that deeply disturbed functionality. We will look at cancer in more detail in Chapter 8 (I have devoted a whole chapter to it as it is such a big area of misunderstanding – and fear – in our misguided medical model).

In this chapter we are going to look at the metabolic disturbances that pre-date such devastating diseases. According to Ari Whitten, health guru and educator, health requires 2 main capacities at a cellular level:

1. Efficient cell regeneration
2. Maintenance of mitochondria (the cellular engine) via autophagy

So we will look at both those in turn, starting with cell regeneration.

Cell Regeneration and Lifestyle Interventions

Efficient cell regeneration (what Dr Robyn Benson calls 'regenerative lifestyle' habits consist primarily of the following factors:

Diet

Here we are talking about eating well (i.e. sufficient wholesome foods, avoiding processed foods – anything with ingredients you don't recognise is likely to be processed) with macronutrients (fats, carbs and proteins) *and* vitamins/minerals). Most people are not eating this way. They eat too many calories with no nutrients – we are truly over-fed and yet undernourished. We also tend to eat more or less continuously throughout the day (grazing and snacking) which never allows our digestive system to rest. And we often eat separately from each other on laps, in cars and at desks without the regulatory processes of conversation, laughter and plenty of chewing!

Eating seasonally

We have learned that we can have the same foods year round because of their general availability in supermarkets but this is not a natural state of affairs. When it's cold outside we need to eat foods that warm us i.e. in winter more soups and roasted vegetables,. Using ginger, garlic and cayenne which also warm us. Then more salads, fruit and cooling foods in summer.

Also eating different rainbow coloured foods each day (with variation) and minimising processed foods and sugar, caffeine, etc allows us to benefit from a variety of phyto-nutrients and keep our microbiome healthy at the same time. Most people eat the same foods each day, and tend to rely on 3 foods as their mainstay: wheat, corn and soy. If you look at the ingredients of most processed foods they will contain variants of these – high fructose corn syrup the ubiquitous sweetener is in virtually everything as it's so cheap and adds sweetness even to savory foods where it is often disguised.

The human body is adapted to foods and not industrialised foodstuffs which have been made in a laboratory not a kitchen.

Sleep Quality and Circadian Rhythm

Sleep is vital for health; good quality sleep particularly. However, that is getting increasingly difficult to achieve in our modern day world. A recent report highlighted that most people were sleep deprived, especially teenagers who require more. So, one aspect that you need to look at is sleep hygiene: keeping your room dark and cool while sleeping.

We have a natural sleep wake cycle and a time when our digestion works best. We could say that there are both circadian and **ultradian** rhythms (those that pass through more than one cycle in a day) in the body – related to solar and lunar cycles. Daytime belongs to the sympathetic system mostly - this is when we move and eat i.e. breakdown things (**catabolism**)[i].

The parasympathetic system is mostly active at night where it activates mitosis (cell division) and regeneration and building of the body (**anabolism**). There is a reason for this; if mitosis was allowed to happen during the day, "radiation could damage the genes so it does it mainly at

---

[i] The Sympathetic system also stimulates apoptosis (pre-programmed cell death and destruction so is basically re-modelling us.

night. So the body is literally a wake, sleep; wake, sleep system; destroy, build, destroy, build; catabolic and anabolic"[61]

Our liver for instance is programmed to do its essential detoxification work at night during the early hours of the morning (usually 2 – 4pm for most people). In addition we are programmed to go to sleep when it is dark and wake when it is light by the action of light on the pineal and the release of melatonin. However a lot of us ignore this idea as we work late into the night or use bright lights (TV, cellphones, blue screens, etc) before bedtimes. Most of us have no idea of the cellular cost of these habits. A cheap solution to this (if you must work late at night!) is to get a red light filter on the screen (f.lux or similar), or a pair of orange-tinted glasses to block out the damaging blue light. Check the internet you'll find lots of options for this. But much better is to time your work to the early morning as it's much more natural to be working in daylight.

The liver also has a **diurnal rhythm** where it expands during the day and shrinks at night (when clearing out toxins – the reverse is true for mice which are active at night). A castor oil pack on the liver during the evening and overnight helps to promote this natural clearance[i].

Reducing our exposure to electromagnetic fields (EMF's) is important for sleep – it reduces our natural melatonin production which affects our immune system and cancer protection. We can do this by at the very least

"turning off your router, or any wireless connectivity device when you are asleep[ii] or add biofield protection to yourself and your devices. EMF's are particularly damaging when the brain is asleep as the electromagnetic wave pattern of the brain alters in sleep and it more closely matches that of electronic devices than when awake. So, if you do nothing else, make sure you keep your bedroom clean of EMFs."

In addition, put your cellphone on airplane mode while carrying it next to your body (in a handbag or rucksack for instance) and switch if off at night (or to airplane mode if you must keep it on) and do not wear fitbits and wearables which communicate via Bluetooth to your cellphone at night. Our quest to know more about our sleep is actually fuelling our insomnia!

---

i Castor oil packing is an old-fashioned but very effective process by which you soak a cloth with castor oil and put it over the liver area with heat. This draws out toxins through the skin.
ii Modern routers recommend not turning them off and on again or they slow the wi-fi signal. So it is probably better to put a biofield protector like a smartdot on them.

This addiction to technology is having huge affects on the quality of our sleep which ultimately determines our health - insomnia and depression are linked[62].

When we go to bed we need to have very little light to sleep well – and this is difficult if we live in a brightly lit city. Internet guru Dr Mercola recommends getting blackout curtains fitted but at the very least sleeping with a cotton or silk eye mask is a simple way of achieving more darkness to the brain. This allows the brain to shrink in order to do its drainage work – where the **glymphatics** (glial cells and lymphatic vessels) are able to drain the lymph fluid with its toxins out of the brain.

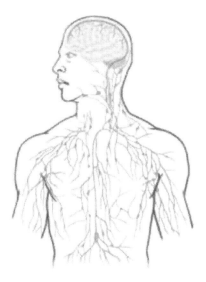

Figure 37: Glymphatics of the Brain

It has been noted that there are seasonal differences in inflammatory markers in the blood and cerebrospinal fluid (CSF); with more pro-inflammatory cytokines present in the winter – up to 30% more! This has profound implications for psychiatric health and may explain some of the reasons behind Seasonal Affective Disorder (SAD)[63]. In modern times we seldom mark the seasons, or notice them in the way we did when we lived and worked on the land.

Movement/ Exercise

We are designed to move. In the past we would have spend most of our waking hours moving. It is only in the last century following the rise of the post-industrial world, that most workers have become sedentary. This has consequences not only at the macro level of muscles and connective tissue, but at a cellular level as we will see.

Exercise is also known to have important mood-altering properties and to be highly beneficial in depression, for instance. It seems to encourage **neurogenesis** (creation of new neurons and neuronal connections) which may be how it combats depression..[64]

However, the type of exercise is really important and needs to be tailored to the person. For instance, for some people: "exhaustive exercise can generate excessive reactive oxygen species (ROS), leading to oxidative stress-related tissue damages and impaired muscle contractility."[65] If you don't work up to it gradually and make sure your diet includes increased amounts of antioxidants (Vitamins C, E, glutathione and CoQ10 amongst others)[66], your body cannot 'mop up' the free radicals and ROS produced in the mitochondria when we exercise.

Recent research has shown that not all exercise is equal. It used to be thought that you would have to do intense cardio-vascular exercise for long periods to get benefit but we now know that intermittent bursts of exercise are actually better. One thing for certain is we were designed to exercise *outdoors* both for Vitamin D production and natural light hormonal stimulation of our sleep/wake cycle. Moderate rather than extreme cardiovascular exercise at least three times a week seems to promote healthy blood flow and it helps mitochondria to renew (mitophagy).

Epigenetic effects of exercise

How it does this is that it changes the signalling inside the cells via the read-out of DNA:

"Exercise is a powerful **epigenetic modifier** i.e. changing your gene expression. This is particularly true if you do some each day (approximately 20 minutes of aerobic exercise per day). Ideally it will be something you enjoy (the answer to the question 'what is the best exercise') but be it doesn't have to be onerous. Burst (interval) training with several 3-4 min aerobic exercise alternating with periods of 'cool down' are most effective - much more so than an hour on a treadmill believe it or not. This is because it boosts human growth hormone (HGH)[i], which despite its name isn't just for our childhood years but an important regulatory 'feel good' hormone throughout life for both men and women, but particularly in adolescence[67].

The importance of exercise for our discussion is that it inhibits inflammatory processes of cognitive decline, joint swelling, cardiovascular clogging, etc. How it does this is to 'upregulate' certain protective molecules and promote the detoxification process within the liver - both of these involve **methylation** which is the addition of a methyl group (CH3) to DNA or other molecules"..

The Importance of Sunlight and Vitamin D

Adequate sun exposure allows our body to make Vitamin D in the skin from sunlight of a certain frequency. **Cholecalciferol** is the inactive hormone made in the skin which is converted via sunlight and a two stage process in the liver and kidneys to the active metabolite. Most people in the western world are highly deficient due to our indoor lifestyles. However, it is difficult even to get enough even if we do go outside as, during the winter months in the northern hemisphere, the wavelengths of light are not sufficient[ii]. Vitamin D isn't even a vitamin! It is in fact a powerful pre-hormone involved in myriad reactions in the body so getting your vitamin D status up to optimum is vital.

Vitamin D Receptor - VDR

Vitamin D has been intensively studied in recent years, mainly due to efforts of Michael Hollick in the US.[68] His recognition that Vitamin D is in fact a steroid pre-hormone (cholecalciferol**)** formed mainly in the skin from cholesterol (and lesser so from diet) means it has been misnamed as the definition of the term 'vitamin' actually refers to something we have to have in our food as we cannot make it ourselves. Skin production is by far the major source – it is a highly efficient process that can make several thousand IU's (International Units) in 10 -20 minutes (depending on skin tone and latitude) compared to food sources which we would need to eat pounds of oily fish (the other main source).

Whether formed in the skin or eaten, it is converted in a two-step process from the inactive form first in the liver then to the kidneys for further

---

[i] HGH is produced in the pituitary and stimulates growth, cellular renewal and regeneration and boosts fat-burning via its adrenaline (epinephrine) release.
[ii] in the UK we only make vitamin D reliably between April and October.

conversion into either the active form (**calcitriol**) or another inactive form depending on need. Calcitriol is the actual hormone that does the work throughout the body but it needs other factors such as heparin sulphate (also formed in the skin) to be usable. This is why simply taking supplements or IV Vitamin D can be more tricky to get right and even dangerous[i] .

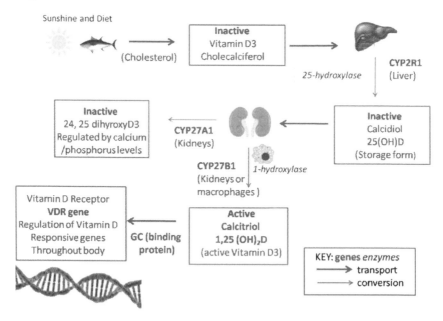

Figure 38: Vitamin D conversion

It used to be thought that Vitamin D was only involved with bone and calcium metabolism (it helps absorb Ca from the gut to put into the bones) until it was found that nearly every cell in the human body has a **Vitamin D Receptor (VDR)**. It is now known to be involved in the cell cycle influencing cell cycling and proliferation, differentiation, and apoptosis. In particular it seems to "influence normal and pathological cell growth, carcinogenesis, immune function, and cardiovascular physiology"[69]. How does it affect the cell in this way? It is a cellular response via a message received on the cell membrane similar to the insulin one we saw earlier.

---

[i] Overdose of Vitamin D is entirely possible this way but impossible through the skin as the body has systems to get rid of excess.

Here it is the VDR which receives the message when Vitamin D docks into it, whereupon it combines with a protein called the RXR to create 3-part molecule called the Vitamin D Response Element (VDRE). This then makes its way to the nucleus to attach to DNA and affect how the DNA is read (i.e. is transcribed into RNA and then proteins). See the diagram below. The VDR seems to be involved in much cell signalling and makes Vitamin D much more than a vitamin.

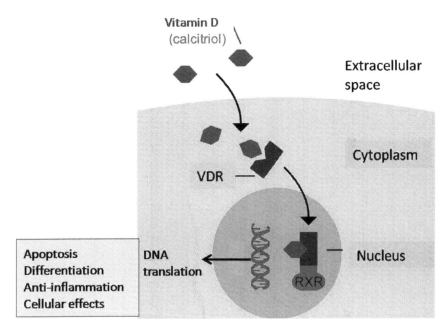

Figure 39: Vitamin D Receptor

Vit D may be involved in cardiovascular health too. The old theory that cardiovascular plaques result from high cholesterol (and homocysteine) may be wrong. A new theory by Stephanie Seneff posits that it is **sulphation** of Vitamin D (addition of a sulphate group to cholecalciferol ChS) and cholesterol in the skin that does the real work. If this is correct (and data seems to corroborate this[70]) the role of ChS is important in red blood cells and in the ECM, including the lining of blood vessels. It has been theorised:

"that heart disease develops in the cardiovascular system as a reaction to deficiencies in critical biosulfates - especially cholesterol sulfate. She suggests that when the body is deficient in sulfates, cardiovascular plaque develops intentionally as an 'alternative mechanism' to make and supply more cholesterol and sulfate to the heart. When sulfate levels are low, artery walls cannot function properly, triggering cascades that lead to plaque production and build-up."

Sulphate deficiency may be 'the biggest deficiency you've never heard of' according to many commentators. Plaques may be "a well-choreographed program for renewal of cholesterol sulfate" in conditions where insufficient dietary sulfur and inadequate sun exposure contribute to low cholesterol sulfate levels"[71]. An intriguing thought.

But daylight doesn't just give us vitamin D. As I said in my first book:

"Infra-red rays restructure water in your body to have a more harmonious electro-chemical structure that mimics the energy of our own body (which is why infra-red (IR) saunas are so good for detoxing). They also make us feel good (summer holidays have this effect not only because of relaxation!). Light helps balance the pituitary too which is the master hormone gland. So, exercising in the sun is better than in the gym. If you are into running, make it a practice to get out in the air not on the treadmill."

Hydration: Drinking Water

We are all being exhorted to drink more water – with snazzily-marketed plastic bottles of vitamin-enhanced water to help us do it. But of course this does not take into account the quality of the water or the additives. Most people do not consider where their water comes from as it is taken for granted that it comes out of a tap[i]. Thus we don't value it and have allowed recycling and sterilisation practices which although giving us 'clean' water[ii] does not necessarily mean good quality. In order to render it potable (drinkable) it has been subject to upwards of 200 chemicals (including trihalomethanes (THMs), bisphosphonates and physical interventions that are far removed from how water would naturally accumulate and be recycled.

"When we were living natural Paleolithic lives we would have obtained our drinking water naturally filtered by rock from natural rainfall (obtained from underground wells or streams). In addition, having moved along a watercourse it would have picked up a lot of positive ions and be 'living' electrochemically-

---

[i] If we had to drink out of streams and rivers we'd be dying at even greater rates than we are. Animals however are not so lucky. 58% of vertebrates have disappeared off the planet since 1970 (WWF). We could be next unless we learn to look after our earth.
[ii] In the UK we have some of the cleanest drinking water on the planet but at a cost.

speaking. Tap water bears no relation to this type of water other than the same chemical signature H$_2$O. Its energetic signature is entirely different[i] ."

In some of the longest-living communities (aka 'Blue Zones') people drink naturally filtered water from wells or springs. Residents of some spa towns in Derbyshire and Yorkshire in the UK can access naturally filtered groundwater, but most of us aren't that lucky and health professionals recommend filtering your tap water e.g. with a reverse osmosis system which fits under the kitchen sink but they are expensive so many people resort to bottled or charcoal filter jugs. There seems no easy solution at the moment unless you happen to be lucky enough to live somewhere where there is natural spring water. but for the rest of us, especially those living in urban environments, this is not possible and we are dependent on bottled or tap water or – largely missed in most articles and books on the subject – mineral-rich water from fruit and vegetables like apples, celery and cucumber. This is naturally filtered water by the plant, if you will. Eating/juicing more of these foods adds significantly to your cellular hydration.

Grounding

Grounding (earthing): rubbing your hands in soil or walking barefoot, for instance. Be in touch with the earth with socks off occasionally – if the weather allows. The surface of the earth has a slight negative electric charge due to its free electron field. Believe it or not grounding - especially walking on the ground with direct contact of your skin - allows you to use these free electrons to balance the positive charge you carry. It is an increasing problem that we don't discharge.

According to the 'father of grounding', Dr Clint Ober, "unfortunately, with our modern rubber or plastic soled shoes and insulated sleeping arrangements, we no longer have a natural electrical connection to the Earth, unless walking barefoot"[ii]. Natural rubber was more conductive as it allowed moisture from our sweat to permeate and therefore the water conducts. Modern plastic-derived rubber is not permeable in the same way.

---

[i] If you find this difficult to believe check the Japanese researcher Masaru Emoto's work on water crystals and human interaction; he found vast differences between those subject to loving vs. hateful thoughts! Interestingly this scientist was a skeptic himself before he did the experiments. See his bestselling book 'The Hidden Messages in Water'.
[ii] See http://www.groundology.co.uk/about-grounding for more information

Thus, we are largely insulated from the earth and now surrounded by positive charge from pollution, including electromagnetic smog, trans fats in our food, and the free radicals produced from metabolic processes (particularly via the immune system which uses them to kill pathogens). These are all stresses on the body. Is it any surprise we are seeing a huge rise in disease as a result?

So how does grounding work? Clint Ober maintains that grounding reduces systemic (system wide) inflammation, the basis of all chronic disease. He further states:

"Inflammatory processes are driven by electron deficient molecules called free radicals or reactive oxygen species (ROS) and these mobile electrons create an antioxidant microenvironment, slowing or preventing ROS) from causing 'collateral damage' to healthy tissue. We also hypothesize that electrons from the Earth can prevent or resolve so-called 'silent or smouldering' inflammation."[72]

Grounding has been demonstrated to reduce inflammation, thin your blood and improve your immune response and shift your nervous system to a parasympathetic state; so called **'vagal stimulation'**. It also changes the viscosity of blood making the blood cells free from clumping; this is huge factor in reducing strokes and heart disease. See the videos by cardiologist Dr. Sinatra and Dr Gupta aka 'York Cardiology' for more information[i].

Why haven't we heard this? Why aren't we told to go outside and earth ourselves or buy an earthing mat for use indoors? The effects are so beneficial and vast[73] that you wonder why you haven't heard it anywhere at your GP's surgery or that the health services like the NHS doesn't subsidise grounding pads for people with chronic illness. I'll leave you to decide but here's a clue – there's no profit in it – most of these interventions are free or very low cost and if everybody did it there would be a reduced need for drugs of all kinds!

However, you can fight back. You can buy grounding devices to connect to your bed so that you ground while you sleep or small pads under your feet or computer while you work too; they plug into a power outlet which fortunately is connected to the earth pin in the electrical plug (I'm using one

---

[i] See https://www.drsinatra.com/ and York Cardiology on Youtube

now while I type!). They bring your voltage down to zero by allowing you to ground to the earth's charge. This is particularly important the higher you sleep above the earth; if you live in a tower block, or flats above the ground your voltage is likely to be even higher[74i]. Note that whenever you are in connection with an electrical device (like your laptop for instance) your voltage rises immediately. You can test this for yourself with a home voltmeter kit. You can get under-bed sheets too. This reduces your voltage to negligible levels which is so important if you work or sleep with electrical equipment around you. If you suffer from hormonal/sleep difficulties this could be something to consider as a simple, fairly low cost method of improving your health. You could say we have an 'electron deficiency syndrome'! It is increasingly the case that most people are disconnected from the earth[ii], which we were never designed to be. Some people are more electrically sensitive than others due to their unique biochemistry.

EMFs and Electrosmog – Threat to Human Health

Don't forget we are electrical beings. We have 3 main electrical systems: the brain, heart and neuroimmunological system (including thyroid). These are important in regulating our biology as much as our biochemistry. DNA and cellular electrolyte balance are particularly vulnerable to damage from electrosmog[iii]. According to Dr Carlos A Ritter, it takes only 30mV to break our DNA and so EMFs may cause problems with both gene regulation and cellular free radical production. Symptoms are many and varied from fatigue and brain fog to headaches and skin issues. Everyone reacts differently which is why it makes it difficult to identify EMFs as the cause.

The main mechanism for the downstream effects appears to be via interference with the **voltage gated calcium channels** which allow a huge influx of calcium into the cell. This triggers a 'slew of negative health effects[75]' . It could be considered an immune sensitivity but to EMFs and largely undiagnosed. Sweden recognises it as a condition but most countries do not. Children, whose brains are still developing, are particularly vulnerable. In Belgium and Switzerland they have recently announced a moratorium to

---

[i] Dr Ritter explores this by measuring household EMFs – explored in his website emfknights.com and Electro-sensitivity UK on www. es-uk.info
[ii] For full info watch the video with Dr Ober and Dr. Mercola on the Groundology website
[iii] Stray electromagnetic radiation from devices permeates our homes and outside environment. See the work of Nick 'The EMF Guy' Pinault

prevent 5G installation until there is more evidence into its safety. Believe it or not there is very little safety testing of this new technology and such that there has been is with limited numbers of people and one device. No-one has yet tested the effects of the mass of exposure from multiple sources that we are now exposed to. The science has been unequivocal for at least 10 years but recent advances in 5G make it much more concerning[76]. See the work of Dr Martin Pall for more info[77,78]. At the very least shield yourself when carrying your cell phone and put onto airplane mode at night. I've covered other options previously.

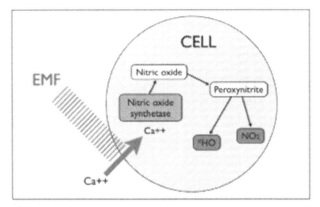

Image Credit: Dr. Paul Dart and Dr. Martin Pall

Figure 40: EMF Activation of Cellular Calcium Channels

Stress reduction

Stress reduction is all of the above interventions (eating well, getting good sleep, reducing our toxin exposure, etc). These are all stresses on the body. But it also includes the more difficult area of dealing with poor relationships, making sure we have meaning and purpose in our lives (a job we do that gives us no joy is profoundly stressful), and engaging with other like-minded people in something that allows us to give to others is also part of the equation. I've dealt with the stress response and techniques for stress alleviation in detail in my first book so won't reiterate it here.

Cellular Recycling - Optimising Autophagy

The final component deserves a longer and more detailed look. Firstly what is autophagy? It is the activity of cellular recycling which allows cells to maintain their health and efficiency. According to Ari Whitten it is to repair the 'junk' that accumulates in the cells "such as malfunctioning mitochondria (our cellular energy generators), misfolded proteins, and other damaged organelles".

This is achieved via the creation of a big bag (auto-phagosome) around the damaged organelle (along with intracellular bacteria and viruses) to isolate and then breakdown the cellular components of that organelle or organism which are then recycled (the proteins are broken down into amino acids that the cell then can reuse).

"Autophagy is normally triggered when our cells are stressed, such as when we are in starvation mode or there is cellular stress from exposure to a toxin. It is considered to be a cytoprotective process.[79]

One of the most important organelles to recycle in order to protect cell function is the mitochondria. Unless we can dispose of old worn out ones, our cells will be poisoned with Reactive Oxygen Species (ROS) (cellular 'rust'). However, too much and there is no capacity within the system. How does the body regulate this process?

This, again, is a process of cellular regulation mediated by a very important peptide called **Insulin-like Growth Factor 1 (IGF-1)**. Under conditions of mild starvation it activates the auto-phagosomes which help to recycle the cell's components. Additionally, autophagy can be directly activated by the kinase network (via mTOR), which we met in chapter 3. Anything we can do to activate IGF production, including most of the activities we've already looked at in this chapter, but in particular intermittent fasting or pulse exercise (aka 'burst training) helps reduce the effects of ageing. We sometimes refer to this as the 'mitochondrial theory of ageing' which we'll cover more in the chapter on Alzheimer's Disease and dementia.

Cellular Detox and the Antioxidant Response Element (ARE)

As commonly understood, 'detoxing' is something you do periodically after a particularly heavy session of eating and drinking (i.e. after Christmas, etc). We have various cultural movements including 'dry January' and Veganuary which attempt to redress this over-indulgence. These procedures are important; fasting was part of tribal man's way of keeping healthy. But they may not be enough to redress the balance in the cell as we constantly over-eat these days, even aside from festivals. Ironically, we end up eating way too much largely to keep the natural detoxification process at bay! Feeling ill is the result of the detox (breakdown or catabolism) itself[i] and eating/drinking is stimulant (build-up or anabolism). As a result our liver (the major the organ of detoxification), is often overwhelmed and cannot maintain optimal cleansing of the blood. This varies too with your genetic predisposition as you may be a fast or slow detoxifier (via CYP gene). When the liver is backed up, our cells begin to get clogged (especially fat cells which tend to store toxins). We need to find ways to enhance our detox capabilities, not just via the liver but at a *cellular* level too.

The balance between anabolism and catabolism in the cell is controlled by certain protein messengers. One of these is the Antioxidant Response Element (ARE), a protein which is produced when activated by a **transcription factor** (something that activates a gene to be read), called Nuclear Related Factor 2 (NRF2)[80]. One way to enhance your ARE is to increase your 'fasting window' – the time between the last meal of the evening and first meal of the day to at least 16 hours. If you struggle with this then make an effort to at least avoid eating 2-3 hours before bed. Detoxing is enhanced in the non-feeding state so we need to have an extended time when we are not digesting.

Excess calories are toxic to brain cells and can cause the 'food crash' (feeling sleepy after food), if not enough antioxidants are present[ii]. It may help to supplement glutathione in this case as it is the body's strongest anti-oxidant. Repair happens about 3 hours after a meal, so we need a prolonged period at night to allow this and reduce our free radical burden. Good sleep is vital for this detox, as are the phyto-nutrients in green veg. But most people need more than this as the toxicity has been going on too long and gone too deeply. A more radical approach may be needed.

Detox Toolkit

According to Dan Pompa, author of True Cellular Detox™, it is the level of neurotoxins in the cell that are a stumbling block for many health-conscious people, who despite eating a good diet and doing regular exercise, are still finding themselves lacking energy and vitality. We are simply overwhelmed with toxins as never before so that the conventional

---

[i] As are migraines – the liver's way of expunging toxins from the liver into the bloodstream
[ii] If this happens to you suspect low antioxidants like glutathione and Vit E or A

approaches may not be enough. He believes "if you don't detox the cell you will never get well."[81] Having undergone his three stage protocol I can report big changes in my health for the better – including being able to sweat again. Many people don't realize that if they have stopped sweating this is not healthy but a sign that the cells are very clogged.

Certainly, toxicity is a big factor in unhealthy ageing and removing those toxins requires patience and a particular protocol that he calls the 'detox toolkit'. Toxins are stored preferentially in the organs that are deemed non-essential by the body (thyroid, spleen, gall bladder and fatty tissue in breast, etc) until eventually the liver and brain may be affected. In order to detox properly you have to draw the toxins out of these organs and boost the elimination pathways (gut, bladder, kidneys, etc) before tackling the deeper organs and cellular structures. You can't just take a detox tea!

The latest supplements that have been developed to enhance cellular detoxification are based on a better understanding of the science of detoxification (often sold as a boost to athletic performance rather than as a solution to chronic illness. My experience of this is that it is very powerful – too powerful for some (including me) and needs to be taken much more slowly by women (whose organs are a third smaller and therefore under more stress) and those who are already suffering from chronic illness. Herbs and plants like chlorella may work for low levels of heavy metals for instance, but for a deeper level of toxicity you need laboratory grade materials that hone in on specific chemicals and draw them out safely via bile (in liver – is often recycled so this can be an issue), urine (kidneys and bladder) and faeces (via gut).

Chapter 6: Ageing and Neuro-degeneration

What is Ageing?

Ageing is not, as commonly assumed, an inevitable process of getting older. It is a process of accumulated damage to cellular mechanisms. In particular, the Mitochondrial Free Radical Theory of Ageing (MFRTA) proposes that it is *accumulated damage to mitochondria* that produces many of the features of ageing. This was proposed as a 'biologic clock' as long ago as 1972 by Harman[82]. The theory has since been extended in more recent research which particularly links it to cancer[83]. We'll cover that in more detail in Chapter 8. First I want to cover some of the general principles.

The process of ageing is not the same in everyone and depends to a large extent on lifestyle i.e. how we live our lives. It can be speeded up or slowed down by what we *do*. Ageing and the diseases of ageing have become synonymous[i] when in fact all disease is a process of *imbalance in the system*. And it will show up in small ways first – these are the 'early warning signs' which we now know are a precursor to more severe illness later on.

For instance migraines may show up from puberty onwards (especially in women). Modern medicine struggles to describe why migraines occur. We know they are linked to excess histamine release causing a sudden relaxation of the blood vessels leading to the brain. Drugs that suppress this response are given to alleviate them but don't deal with the underlying problem as they are *downstream* of the real cause. From a functional/holistic perspective, chronic migraines are the body's attempt at *mobilising toxins for removal*[ii]. Drugs that suppress the migraines only keep it going.

---

[i] Most people now assume that they will die of a disease rather than of 'natural causes'
[ii] I always felt 'lighter inside by the end of my migraine. I now recognise this as my liver having cleared my blood of toxins

Also considered common are conditions of varicose or spider veins, 'red eye', haemorrhoids, chilblains, etc which many people suffer from and are all linked to toxicity in the circulatory system. These are not normal signs of ageing and need to be seen for the warning that they are. I had all these problems in my thirties (yes that young) and don't have them now because I have addressed the nutritional deficiencies by modifying my diet and lifestyle to suit my genetic predisposition.

When I had my gene profile (DNA) read in 2016[i] it became apparent I don't detox well; I had both problems with Vitamin B12, folate and Vitamin A conversion. Everyone has certain minor base pair mutations called **Single Nucleotide Polymorphisms (SNiP s**that make a slight difference in the protein they code for. These epigenetic SNiPs are adaptive in the right circumstances but have become a problem in today's toxic world. With the right supplementation I can tailor my diet with certain nutrients that are rich in the missing compounds my body needs.

Other signs of ageing are liver spots – darkened patches on the skin (usually areas exposed to light like the face and hands) which gradually spread on the skin. This is a signal that your liver is struggling; it is a chemical reaction of AGE's in the skin reacting with sunlight. It is normal in your eighties and nineties but if you have them before this then take it your liver needs support. Your doctor will have no answer to this. They don't learn about nutrition and only deal with illness and outright organ failure not the gradual accumulation of dysfunction or the preventative methods that everyone can undertake. I dealt with solutions to this via bitter herbs and more formal liver detox protocols in my second book so won't repeat here. But take these signs as the warning they are - if your car warning light was flashing you would need to do something! Don't ignore your body – it's your vehicle for life.

Epigenetic Control of Cellular Repair

Cellular health is a direct function of how well metabolic regulation of the competing growth and repair (anabolic) and breakdown (catabolic) mechanisms is operating i.e. the balance of those two opposing processes. This is largely controlled at the cellular level by epigenetic regulation by the neurological, immune and endocrine systems we have already covered.

---

[i] I got my genes read by 23andme. It was revelation. Other companies also do it.

Telomeres and DNA

There is another mechanism used to regulate cellular division and repair called telomeres. The name **telomere** comes from the word for 'the last part' in Greek. It is a sheath or cap around the end of the chromosome which is not copied upon mitosis (cell division). They were discovered by scientists in 2009 – for which they won the Nobel Prize in physiology and medicine.[84] For a long while it was not understood what the function could be; it was noted that they got shorter over time and once the length drops to a certain threshold, the DNA becomes vulnerable to being damaged by ROS (free radicals) in the environment. They are a **biomarker** for ageing so considerable research around how to extend telomere length and thus extend lifespan and prevent premature ageing has ensued.

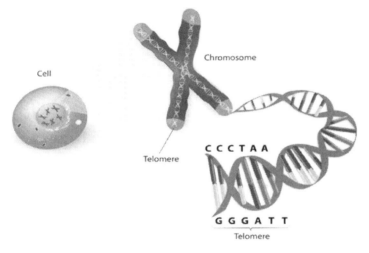

Figure 41: Telomeres

Telomerase enzyme, which repairs damaged telomeres, decreases in function over time, depending on lifestyle factors such as diet, childhood history[i], etc. It is activated by Vascular Endothelial Growth Factor (VEGF)[85] which responds in particular to exercise of a certain type – intense bursts are the best for this (sometimes called interval training). If early childhood was less than supportive, the levels of VEGF are much reduced and obesity and chronic disease often result. Repair requires energy and thus

---

[i] It is an interesting fact that premature babies (who are not held or cuddled by being put in an ICU shortly after birth) develop shorter telomeres and thus accelerated ageing

mitochondrial involvement so there is less protection by damaged mitos. And when telomeres get short certain diseases become more likely: obesity or cancer for instance.

Lifestyle Factors

There are many lifestyle factors that ameliorate threats in your gut flora through epigenetic effects. Modifiable lifestyle factors are one way we can overcome the threat of disease – even the most feared of modern diseases cancer and, especially, the auto-immune type diseases - both of which we are losing the battle with currently. These chronic inflammatory diseases are testing our health services in unprecedented ways that we simply don't have treatments for.

There has been a growing recognition that lifestyle might have something to do with this rise in **non-communicable disease (NCD)** – sometimes just referred to as 'chronic' disease. A return to a primal lifestyle has been mooted as a solution; also known as the 'Paleo' movement. It has been billed as being primarily about changing what you eat but, in fact, is not all about diet. It takes in exercise/outdoor engagement, relationships and connection, managing stress and so on. We need to get back to lifestyles more conducive to health and out of chronic disengagement with our place in the planetary ecosystem. Primitive man had instinctively and it gave his life meaning.

Food, exercise and stress are some of the most powerful epigenetic modifiers; food being the most powerful.. We look at each of these in turn.

Fasting

From the work of Dr Valter Longo, there has been an interest in how modifications to diet, can improve longevity[86]. A recent book, based on interviews with centenarians, outlines a fasting mimicking diet. Undoubtedly an attractive concept that with the right foods at the right time you don't need to fast at all!

Detoxification and Rebuilding the Gut

We are surrounded by chemicals in the air, water and foods that we eat, most of them untested on humans and of dubious safety. Our natural detoxification processes (mostly in the liver) are likely to be overwhelmed. What can we do?

You may have been on detox regimes to help clear the body. These are good, but they only last as long as your regime. How do you make changes that last? Well, the good news is that Lactobaccillus species helps both to break down *and* to help the body break down heavy metals in the diet and eliminate them in the stool. So, adding these to your gut flora is a good start in detoxification and if you create the right conditions for them to proliferate you will have a longer term solution to the problem of heavy metals. Unfortunately, if you have ever had a dose of broad spectrum antibiotics (as most of us have) you are likely to have lost the diversity of your gut flora, and lactobacillus being one of the most prolific in the large intestine, is likely to have been denuded.

Disease is a systemic breakdown, a sign of poor maintenance not a random failure of individual organs or glands. This is really the difference in outlook between natural (holistic) and conventional views of health. We must support the weakest point in the system which is causing its failure; this is actually a common understanding in engineering just not in medicine!

Supporting the Mitochondria

If you have a chronic illness, you might need to also support the mitochondria in the cell to allow toxins to come out of the extra-cellular membranes to be cleared out, via the liver and blood. You can't rush the process and you must respect your body's integrity and natural way of doing things. Those who rush into detoxification, may initially feel good when they clear out, but the issue will come back when they don't support the body properly. Also, if they have adrenal fatigue issues (as chronic stress tends to encourage), detoxification itself will be identified by the body as a threat and you will feel worse[87]. Some call this the Herxheimer reaction. Don't forget, to reduce inflammation in the cell membrane you will need anti-oxidants and chelators (pronounced key-late-ors) to neutralise those toxins (both internal metabolic waste and environmental toxins like mercury). To support your mitochondria:

1. Reduce inflammation (removing parasites and other sources)
2. Repair cell membranes (omega-3 fats)
3. Boost ATP energy production

4.   Provide Vitamin B/folate methyl donors – transmutates (neutralises) toxins and repairs DNA
5.   Repair free radical damage. Provide anti-oxidants e.g. Selenium for Super-oxide dismutase (SOD - one of the free radical repairing enzymes) and glutathione as supplements
6.   Re-build gut the flora

You have to work to this level of clearance if you want to live a long and healthy life. As Dr Jack Tips says, "we live and die at the cellular level" and this is a profound truth.

Thyroid Sensing and Health

Thyroid health is so important and often missed; a lot of mothers are low in thyroid hormone (hypothyroid) when they give birth (linked to the necessary shift in immune response from Th1 to Th2 to prevent rejection of the baby). Thyroid hormone is an iodine-containing molecule which helps us produce energy, amongst other things. People with low thyroid often feel sluggish and low in energy and 'joie de vivre'. They feel horrible in fact. Recent studies have pointed to an alarming increase in hypothyroidism in western nations, with women much more affected than men[i]. Official statistics say that prevalence is around 2% of the UK population but significant figures, like Dr Thierry Hertoghe, President of the International Hormone Society, a respected physician's organisation, suggest the real figure may be 20% to 50% of a standard population[ii].

Thyroid health is intricately linked to the brain-heart-gut axis and a more masculine energy (Type A or driven/over-thinkers) who also happen to be highly sensitive (HSP). This means they get drained easily (as they tend to perceive stress more) and get energetically imbalanced. It is also linked to conservation of resources in time of perceived threat. For instance, did you know that the Irish have a higher incidence of Hashimoto's thyroiditis because their epigenetic message of scarcity (from the Irish potato famine) has survived in their genes to slow their metabolism more. According to Isabella Wentz "this is because in time of famine, it's really important for us

---

[i] Hypothyroidism is mostly seen in women ten times more than men and tending to be between the ages of 40 - 50.
[ii] Hypothyroidism is often missed by doctors using outdated reference ranges. According to Dr Kellman, most hypothyroidism is due to toxic chemicals that act as endocrine disruptors. But the story is more complex than that even, with trauma and stress playing a big part.

to conserve our resources." It makes perfect sense but in today's world of excess calories and excess stress it doesn't help us quite so much.

The thyroid is also part of the innate immune system (primarily in the gut). As Wentz further states:

"The innate immune response is known to be triggered when the thyroid gland becomes infected by a pathogen, like the Epstein-Barr virus, or when it is damaged by radiation or another toxin. The damage to the tissue releases molecules that call out to the immune system to help clear the pathogens, damaged cells, and begin cell repair. These molecules (DAMPs that we saw in Chapter 3), can initiate and perpetuate an inflammatory response within a tissue or an organ as the cells that are sent in may further damage thyroid cells.[88]"

We must understand the thyroid is a sensing organ that picks up and perpetuates danger signals in our environment which helps us determine whether we are safe or not. Then it triggers an autoimmune response as part of the immune signalling of danger[i]. We know that women have a greater variability of immune response due to being more vulnerable in society in general and, more specifically, being responsible (largely) for bringing new life into the world. In order to carry a child they need to be:

"particularly tuned into sensing the environment to make sure that the time is prime for reproduction. After all, pregnancy is a huge stress on the body that requires resources. If you are in a situation where resources are scarce, it's generally easier to survive if you're not pregnant. As infertility is a side effect of thyroid disease, perhaps the immune system attack on the thyroid gland is an effort to help us survive.[89]"

It makes perfect sense, then, that the vast majority of sufferers of thyroid disorders are women. It is part of what has been termed '**adaptive physiology**'. If they do get pregnant however, the implications for the child and mother are huge. The baby's brain needs a good supply of the thyroid hormone T4 (converted in the body to the active hormone T3). So a low value in the pregnant mother is significant for the brain development of their child. Spontaneous miscarriage may be linked to the adaptive shift failure whereby the T4/3 levels are not able to rise enough and the immune system rejects the baby. If the body isn't able to regenerate the thyroid post-

---

[i] People who have been abused or traumatised have lifelong changes in their thyroid hormones with decreased levels of active thyroid hormone T3

partum then post-natal depression is very likely. Often this is the first time that thyroid disease is identified. PND is common in the first few months but normally rights itself as the immune system switches back to its normal balance.

Firstly, according to Aviva Romm, MD, thyroid hormone affects breast-milk production, energy, mood and the ability to be present with the child.[90] As I described in my last book in more detail, a child learns emotional regulation from the interaction with their mother. An absence of connection, termed 'attachment' in psychology, has lifelong consequences for the nervous system balance of that child. It makes them hyper-reactive to stress, as we have already described.

Neuro-degeneration and Ageing

We have unfortunately conflated ageing and neurodegenerative disease as the same thing so that we regard it almost normal to become demented with old age. This is far from the truth. Dementias like Alzheimer's and Parkinson's are *disease states of the brain and nervous system* and have little to do with normal ageing other than they tend to co-occur because of a gradual failure of the restorative functions of the cell.

Neurodegenerative disorders (diseases of damage to the nervous or neurological system) of all types are on the rise. According to researchers, metabolic dysfunction, oxidative stress and neuro-inflammation lie at the heart of these diseases:

"Neurons are among the most metabolically active cells in the body, requiring the correct balance of oxygen and glucose to maintain healthy function. However, when the metabolic balance is overwhelmed and the sum of free radicals in a cell is greater than the capacity of the cell to detoxify these substances, oxidative stress is generated. Increased oxidative stress has been shown to contribute to the etiology or progression of a number of neurodegenerative diseases since the brain uses a disproportionate amount of oxygen per volume of tissue compared to other organs [1]. When free radicals of oxygen are present within the environment of the cell, they may damage lipid membranes, interfere with DNA integrity, and interrupt cellular respiration through alterations in mitochondrial complex I (of the electron transport chain).[91]"

Neuro-inflammation and the Brain - Insulin Resistance

How does that translate into the problems we see in neurodegenerative disease? Well, it's an interesting fact that two-thirds of the brain actually consists of white matter (constituting helper or **glial cells)** compared to a third grey matter (neurons or nerve cells). There are three types of glial cells with the most important for our discussion being the **microglial** (immune) cells. Further, when we consider that neurons and immune cells possess *the same receptors* for brain-derived neuropeptides,[92] which signal the state of the organism, then clearly neuro-inflammation – the primary way that the immune system attacks a threat - is going to be very significant. It has been said that neurodegenerative disease is primarily a sign of auto-immunity (attack of the self). According to Harvard researcher Datis Kharrazian, "most of the chronic neurodegenerative diseases of our time are a consequence of neuro-inflammation and immunological activity."[93]

Most chronic disease is inflammatory in nature, even heart disease and diabetes. Recently Alzheimer's Disease (AD) has been added to the canon as it has been found to have an important inflammatory component, due to our carb-heavy diets making brain cells insulin resistant just like in diabetes. For this reason, it has recently been given the name 'Type 3 Diabetes' to reinforce this link.[94] With an altered glucose metabolism, brain cells become resistant to insulin as much as those in the body do. This is primarily because the receptors on the cell surface become less sensitive to the insulin which would normally control the blood sugar level. Continual high blood sugar is dangerous to the body and the body responds with release of messengers called cytokines. With these resulting high levels of circulating inflammatory cytokines (called the **inflammasome** by researchers), mitochondria are poisoned so they become less efficient. This affects the cardiovascular (blood), lymphatic and endocrine systems and damage occurs to the blood supply to the brain too, further restricting its metabolism. It's a downward cycle of degradation.

Fat and the Brain

So what of the specific effect on brain cells? The brain is a metabolically hungry organ; it primarily uses glucose for fuel to preserve its fatty structure[i].

Fat is very important to the brain both structurally and functionally i.e. to insulate the neurones with their myelin sheath (the fatty insulator around the nerve fibre). The maintenance of the myelin sheath is the job of the **astrocytes**[i], another form of glial (helper) cells. But for this it needs a plentiful supply of good fats.

The brain has to be protected from microbial infection and oxidation of its fats. It uses the ability of the lipoproteins to transfer lipids (small fats) and cholesterol across the blood-brain barrier in a carefully controlled manner. Fat cannot normally be transported dissolved in watery liquids like blood (fat and water do not mix and they would be damaged by oxygen), so instead it is bundled into spherical package with proteins called **lipoproteins**. You many have heard of these as 'good' (**Low Density Lipoproteins - LDL**) or bad 'cholesterol' (**High Density Lipoproteins - HDL**) but this is a strange mistelling of the story (to suit the selling of statins by the pharmaceutical industry).

Firstly these describe not the cholesterol itself (which is a necessary and essential fatty molecule for heart and brain function) but *the way they are transported around the body* i.e. the lipoproteins. These vary in size depending on how much fat and cholesterol they contain. See diagram below:

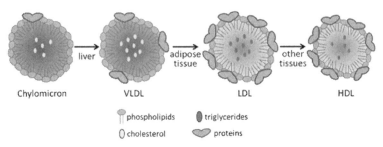

Chylomicron = delivery of fats and cholesterol to liver from gut
VLDL = very low density lipoprotein (high fat) – absorbed in gut
IDL = intermediate density liprotein (moderate fat) – not shown
LDL= low density lipoprotein (low fat) delivered to fat cells for storage 'bad'
HDL – high density lipoprotein (very low fat – delivered to tissues including brain 'good'

Figure 42: Lipoprotein Types and Function

---

[i] A baby's brain uses about 90% of its energy to help it develop. Ketones have historically been found to be a preferential fuel on a low-carb diet.
[i] Astrocytes outnumber neurons 3:1 so are an incredibly important part of the brain

The body conserves cholesterol as it is precious cargo – it is about 90% recycled in the liver from bile. The brain needs to be able to import this from the circulating blood supply but without importing *damaged* cholesterol. This is done by lipoproteins of different sizes as shown above. With an excess of circulating glucose (which insulin would normally reduce), proteins in the brain become damaged as we have already described elsewhere in the body. The protein plaques and tangles[i] that were previously thought to be the cause of Alzheimer's are there not to damage the brain but to protect the damage from going further.

Genetic Predisposition and ApoE lipoproteins

So we have seen that the symptoms of poor cellular detoxification are at the heart of why the body ages prematurely and degrades. Disease is the natural result of this clogging. But the body is able to compensate for a long time, which is why disease may not strike immediately, but 30 – 40 years down the line. This is made more or less likely by the interplay with our genes – some genes are particularly implicated in cellular dysfunction. One of those particularly related to blood sugar control is the ApoE4 SNiP (single nucleotide polymorphism or one base substitution in the DNA). This codes for a blood protein called apolipoprotein which carries cholesterol around in the blood. You can inherit different versions of this SNiP which affects which lipoprotein you express. ApoE2 is highly efficient and gives you an advantage (but it's rare), ApoE3 is the default average efficiency protein and ApoE4 present in 13-15% of the population, is the allele (variant) that is associated with increased risk of Alzheimer's.

Table 2: Apoliprotein SNiP and Alzheimer's Risk

Allele	Efficiency of transport	Risk of AD
ApoE2	Highly efficient	Low risk
ApoE3	Average efficiency	Moderate
ApoE4	Low efficiency	High risk

Much has been written about this to scare people that if they have this particular gene SNiP they are much more likely to get neurodegenerative

---

[i] These abnormal deposits show up in brain tissues- revealed by scans and dissection staining.

disease. However, this is a misunderstanding – it is a higher predisposition *only if you do nothing.* With an understanding and a change of lifestyle, much can be done to reduce your risk. According to Stephanie Seneff:

"ApoE plays a critical role in the transport of cholesterol and fats to the brain, it can be hypothesized that insufficient fat and cholesterol in the brain play a critical role in the disease process. In a remarkable recent study, it was found that Alzheimer's patients have only 1/6 of the concentration of free fatty acids in the cerebrospinal fluid compared to individuals without Alzheimer's"

So if you increase your good fats towards a high fat/ low carb diet, you can reverse your natural tendency by increasing essential fats in the brain.

Blood Brain Barrier

There is a special feature of the brain called the 'blood-brain barrier' (BBB), "an extensive three-dimensional interface between the brain and the blood vessels carrying material from the rest of the body for selective exchange of information."[95] It also has the important function of keeping out toxins from vital processes of the brain. It has many similarities to the lining of the gut in that it is a single layer of endothelial cells supported by a basement membrane. Just like the gut, the **tight junctions** between basement cells are controlled by various cytokines to be *selectively permeable* to keep out bacteria, unwanted immune cells and toxins. Selective transporters are also present for important cytokines like leptin influence appetite and satiety.

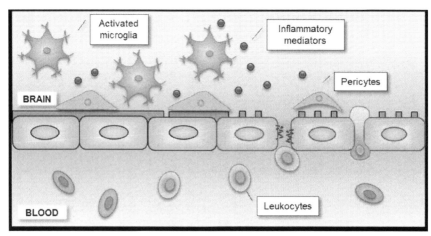

Figure 43: Blood-Brain Barrier

128

Indeed, it used to be thought that the brain was sterile, but we now know that isn't true. It does have bacteria but they are limited by the BBB to maintain balance. But with a poor microbiome, the BBB becomes leaky just like the gut barrier, so the brain becomes bathed in higher levels of glucose than is good for it. Hence, the best preventative solution, in addition to healing the gut of course, is restricting your sugar intake i.e. more eating of *slow-releasing* carbohydrates and more protein/fat. This is the single most important preventative action you can take in your middle age years - before disease strikes you. But there are other interventions which may help us identify and manage this disease.

New types of MRI/EEG are so sophisticated that they can measure levels of glutathione in the brain; a protective, anti-oxidant chemical which scavenges free radicals throughout the body (and brain). Recent studies have shown that this oxidative stress process is part of the pathology of AD (as in diabetes – it could be considered diabetes of the brain[96]) and that low glutathione levels might be implicated in its development[97]. This raises hope for earlier detection as glutathione might be considered a possible biomarker for AD[98]. In other words, the presence of low values of glutathione might be considered an early warning sign of high AD risk. However, as usual, there is much hyperbole around the issue and the politics of how to increase your glutathione have even raged around increased dairy in the diet with some people recommending this. I personally would question that finding – dairy milk, on the whole, is not a natural food anymore given its production and adulteration with hormones.

Smell as a Biomarker of Cognitive Decline

According to Dr Tom O'Bryan, because the olfactory (smell) centres go straight to the brain (bypassing the blood-brain barrier), any defect in the sense of smell acts as a biomarker of inflammation in your brain. Thus it acts as an early warning sign if you are losing your sense of smell[99]. It is a breach of the blood brain barrier or 'B4' as it has been termed. All the diseases of ageing and the diseases that precede it – depression, anxiety, etc come from a problem with B4. Lack of smell can also be a problem with low zinc (as well as brain inflammation generally) and lack of zinc is linked with the development of dementia so there are large correlations.

Metabolic View of Neuro-degeneration

You will have understood from Chapter 2 that I don't consider chronic disease as separate entities in the way modern medicine does. A systems view shows us that many diseases have common components of mitochondrial dysfunction and inflammation – particularly diseases of ageing such as we are considering here. What could be causing this pandemic of chronic inflammatory disease? We have to look again at what is happening in the cell to poison or disable the mitochondria. Could deficiency be at play?

K2 & Mitochondria

Vitamin K was discovered and named in 1929 by a German scientist Heinrich Dam who noticed its propensity to facilitate blood coagulation or koagulation in German – hence the 'K'. Now we know there are two forms of the vitamin: Vitamin K1 (the blood clotting factor - **phylloquinone**) found in leafy greens and **Vitamin K2 (menaquinone - MK)** found in fermented foods especially natto (a Japanese fermented condiment). Vitamin K2 (with Vitamin D3) is now known to be involved in both bone metabolism and arterial health and recent discoveries make it perhaps the greatest secret in maintaining cardiovascular health too.

However, a new role of K2 in mitochondrial energy production is coming to light. Mitochondria are significant in nerve health, because along with muscle contraction and cardiac and brain function, nervous transmission and repair are energy-hungry activities. So we would be unsurprised to find that when our mitochondria are not functioning well, neither are our nerve cells.

We know that bacteria produce K2 (hence their presence in fermented foods) and that Bacillus species especially use them for what is called a **redox** function (reduction/oxygenation – the adding and removal of oxygen or the removal /adding of Hydrogen (H_2) ions when recycling K2. This process takes place within the mitochondria via the Electron Transport Chain (ETC) to produce the energy we need for functioning via the 'energy currency' of ATP (See Chapter 2)

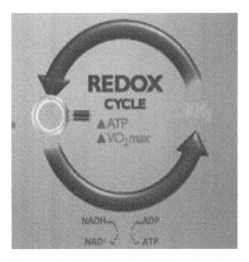

Figure 44: Simplified ATP Production

Vitamin K2 increases the efficiency of the process by its ability to recycle the ATP (which acts as an **electron carrier)**. This often is the rate-limiting step (slowest point) for this form of aerobic respiration. K2 is even better than CoQ10 at rescuing mitochondrial function so *must be taken by anyone suffering from chronic disease of any kind.*

It may even be able to reverse neurodegenerative diseases like Parkinson's Disease (PD) and **Multiple Sclerosis (MS)** – I discuss uses in specific diseases later in this chapter. But for healthy people, especially athletes who demand a lot of their heart and muscles, it is important to dose with K2 as it increases efficiency of mitos by 12% in 8 weeks! It also reduces cramping of muscles as it antagonises (competes for) acetylcholine, the neurotransmitter of contraction. Finally it is arguably the *most important anti-*[100]*a geing nutrient* as it increases mito efficiency and reduces oxidative damage by excessive production of free radicals or 'ROS' and thus mitochondrial death. This Mitochondrial Free Radical Theory of Ageing has already been touched upon. The efficiency of mitochondria is what makes the cell die when it drops to a certain threshold. So by increasing your K2 you improve all the functions of the body that require energy (that's everything!)

Fermented foods

Recent research has shown us the importance of the microbiome in health and wellbeing. I talked about this extensively in my last book The World within. I lamented the loss of fermented foods in our diet that has huge repercussions for the *diversity* of our microbiome. Recent research has shown that the Korean fermented food kimchi may inhibit the degeneration of the mitochondria that is at the heart of neuro-degeneration. Not just because of the vitamin K2 made by the bacteria it contains but more directly as it helps to reinvigorate the mitochondrial degradation that is at the heart of the disease.

Mitochondrial Signalling

How mitochondria adapt to conditions inside the organism is particularly key to neuro-degeneration. We have looked in detail at how mitos produce energy through electron transport (ETC) and the redox cycle. But this understanding only considers *individual* mitos. We need to understand that, just like bacteria, they *live in communities* within the cell. They are not isolated as single organelles as the diagrams in Chapter 2 may have indicated. They are continually interacting with each other: When conditions are right they fuse to form guilds to better produce energy, when conditions are poorer they split to form small vesicles which are then disposed of.

This is termed the **fission/fusion cycle** and it involves a complex array of enzymes and DNA fragments to control. Mitochondrial capacity to produce energy is related to their age and the accumulated damage to their very sensitive enzyme complexes by oxidation (remember 'rust' or ROS?). Excess production of these is what we mean by oxidative damage. Mitochondrial enzyme systems (aka the electron transport chain- ETC) are very sensitive to damage from excess reactive oxygen species like ROS). When they no longer function well, the signalling molecules like ATP and **AMP (Adenosine monophosphate** - ATP minus 2 phosphate groups) indicate to the cell that they need to divide so that the damaged mitos can be disposed of by mitophagy (eating by **phagocyctosis** in the lysosome), the parts recycled to then form new mitos by biogenesis. This cycle takes about 20 minutes in a neuron. See the diagram below for a quick summary.

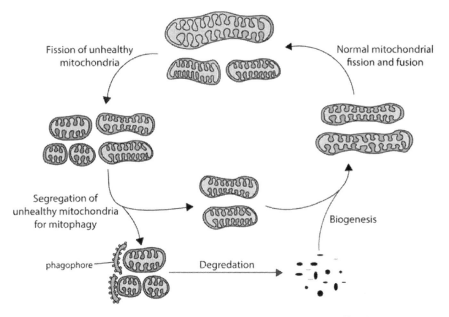

Figure 45: Mitochondrial Fission and Fusion Cycle

It really is fascinating. Here again it helps to understand their bacterial origins as this is exactly what bacteria do to rapidly multiply and thus survive. This adaptation is particularly important in neurons (nerve cells). According to Jon Lieff MD:

"mitochondria respond instantly to mental processes and provide the fuel for all activities of the neuron — buffering calcium signals that determine axon firing and transmission of neurotransmitters; movement of vesicles providing material to the far-flung spaces of the neuron; building and altering structures for neuroplasticity; the electrical spike along the axon; the metabolism that builds proteins, lipids and steroids; and the assembly and movement of the structural tubules. Mitochondria are also vital to the quality control system for the entire cell including programmed cell death. Mitochondria must adapt to each of these tasks, multiply and move into the proper locations. While spawned near the cell body, mitochondria travel throughout the entire cell including axons that are two feet long."

It is important to understand that fusion and division are opposing forces operating all the time. It is the *balance* that dictates cellular efficiency – if more degradation (fission – leading to mitophagy) occurs, then the cell will be low energy-producing. If more **biogenesis** (fusion) occurs, then the cell is going to be higher in output. It constitutes a regulatory mechanism for energy efficiency. Many brain diseases have defects in the ability of mitochondria to fuse, divide, make energy, or deal with stress.[101] Lack of mitochondria also affects muscle strength so plays a large role in the ongoing weakness of muscles with ageing. Given that one of the biggest causes of death in the elderly is hip fracture during a fall, it's worth noting that it's not just because the bones are weak. When the muscle strength is low, the fall becomes inevitable as the person can't hold themselves up.

Mitochondria in Neurons

Nerve cells need a lot of energy due to their transmission of the nerve signal over long distances and through complex networks. The **action potential** is the electrochemical signal that passes down and it is propagated largely by mitochondria. In particular, mutations in fusion genes in humans cause neurodegenerative diseases because mitos become less efficient metabolically when they form smaller vesicles. Fusion dilutes the mutations that may be less beneficial and allows a network to be established which can share information. It also affects the speed of movement along the axon; when they need to move along the cell they do so more efficiently when fused. The microtubules that we met in Chapter 3 are the 'tracks' along which these fused mitos move.

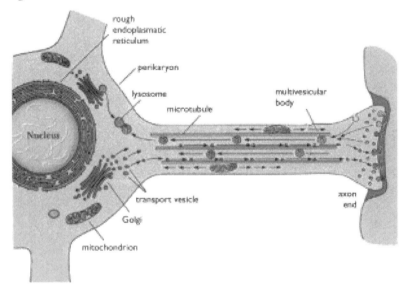

Figure 46: Mitochondrial Transport in Neurons

So how do mitos move along neurons? According to Dr Jon Lieff:

"neurons have a unique protein, **syntaphilin**, that binds to the mitochondrial outer membrane and immobilizes mitochondria in particular locations. It brakes various motors along the mitocrotubules and then becomes a scaffolding molecule to stabilize the mitochondria where energy is needed. When this is completed, syntaphilin rearranges and re-starts the motility..[102]

So this protein is like a scaffolding that is put up and then taken down to allow the movement to continue. Amazing isn't it when we look inside the cell like this rather than as a static picture?

With the understanding that all diseases have similar starting points (inflammation and metabolic changes to mitochondria) but may play out differently in people according to genetic susceptibility and environment, we turn our attention to the most common neurodegenerative diseases and specific understandings in the next Chapter.

Chapter 7: Neurodegenerative Diseases

We have seen in the previous chapter the basis of neuro-degeneration is toxicity and inflammation. Now we turn to the specific diseases of this process – though noting the fact that despite modern medicines treatment of these as separate entities, their precursors are very similar.

Alzheimer's Disease and Dementia

Alzheimer's Disease (AD) is, perhaps secondary to cancer, our most feared disease. Due to its progressive loss of function and deterioration of memory and personality, it can seem to those of us watching it happen to our loved ones, like a slow death. However, it is very important to understand it is NOT inevitable or a genetic disease (except for early onset dementia which accounts for around 2 – 3% of cases); it is a *metabolic* disease, brought about by epigenetic (lifestyle) phenomena – and thus reversible and preventable – despite what the medical establishment tells you. Moreover this is especially important for women who show a 2:1 propensity. There are various theories for this maybe due to their larger hormonal variation – mostly around menopause when oestrogen and progesterone rapidly declines. Whatever the cause, there is an alarming 630% increase in prevalence in women in the last 20 years[i].

The disease is characterised by brain shrinkage, an increase in protein mis-folding and aggregation – most particularly a peptide (small protein) called **amyloid beta (Aβ)**[ii] which is deposited in the roughly 100 trillion neurons of the brain. Let's look at what happens at the synapse in this case. Remember, this is the gap between neurons where the information

---

[i] According to research Dietrich Klinghardt MD
[ii] It is in fact a form of glycation like AGE's we talked about before. Excess sugars attach to the protein making it not fold properly and become 'sticky. Another similarity to diabetes.

(neurotransmitters and peptides) are transmitted across the gap. Aβ is one such neuropeptide and is normally cleared away by the microglial cells which can be thought of as the 'janitors' of the brain[103]. They do their clearance at night when we are asleep but for various reasons, including poor sleep and insulin resistance, sometimes the clearance doesn't happen and Aβ begins to accumulate in the gap where it forms sticky clumps called **amyloid plaques**.

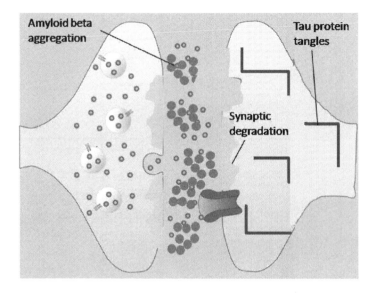

Figure 47: Brain Synapse Degradation with Amyloid & Tau Proteins

Once the plaques have reached a certain 'tipping point' where the aggregations are sufficiently dense, the synapse itself begins to degrade and other **tau proteins** begin to form along the neuronal axon (extensions). These can be clearly seen in the brain of people suffering from this disease.

These mis-folded proteins are far from a normal part of ageing, but *the brain's attempt to deal with the toxicity* which has accumulated over the lifespan – a bit like cholesterol does in the cardiovascular system. It may involve cell signalling with transcription factor NFkB which seems to encourage protein misfolding and neuro-inflammation. The process is degenerative because once started it tends to be progressive. At least that is what has been believed by medicine which is working on a model of the body that is about

100 years out of date and looks at symptoms not causes[i]. Now I want to dive a little bit deeper into the reason that amyloid begins to form. It makes no sense that the body would destroy itself for no reason.

According to expert researcher Dale Bredesen, a new understanding is that amyloid is a *protective protein* that is used by the brain cells to defend against multiple insults to selectively downsize the neuronal response. You won't hear this anywhere in conventional medicine and it is shocking but perhaps understandable therefore that the drugs that have so far been designed are largely useless. Dr Bredesen is at the leading edge of a more holistic view and has designed a programme to reverse cognitive decline in Alzheimer's,[104] He defines 3 main types of AD[ii]:

1. Inflammatory - related to the ApoE4 gene and how our blood sugar balance is dealt with. Those who are pre-diabetic or insulin resistant are more likely to have this.
2. Atrophic - absence of nutrients needed to nurture and supply the neurons e.g., zinc, B_{12}, magnesium, vit D, BDNF, thyroxine
3. Toxic – toxins in the neuron especially metals like mercury, rhino-sinal (nose and sinus) pathogens like Herpes simplex and P. gingivalis and mycotoxins from fungi (often also living in the nose but also breathed in from external sources)[iii] are common sources.

Amyloid is formed from an **amyloid precursor protein (APP)** that needs to be chopped up into smaller bits to become active. . Enzymes act on the APP and cut it into protein fragments, one of which is beta-amyloid (Aβ) and it is crucial in the formation of senile plaques in Alzheimer's. These function as a 'molecular switch' so that the nerve cell can either go in a trophic (synaptoblastic or synapse-building) direction or it can be cleaved to go in an atrophic (synaptoclastic or synapse-destroying) direction. This is much like bone cells which are constantly being made and destroyed. Just like as in osteoporosis in bone, in neurones it is the *balance* between these

---

[i] This old view is still being promulgated by universities in their research– researching for this book I did online training on Alzheimer's and it had no explanation for why just how.
[ii] I would suggest that this relates to the dominant presentation and most people would have all three processes going on to some degree
[iii] Scientists are only just recently beginning to characterise this rhino-sinal microbiome. This along with the gut microbiome is essential.

two activities that dictate how well neuronal connections will be maintained. Amyloid binds divalent metals like mercury, iron and copper which can be in excess; it is therefore *protective to the body* and just getting rid of the protein like many drugs do, actually makes the problem worse!

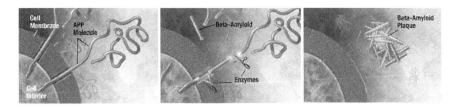

Figure 48: Cleaving of Amyloid to form Plaques

synaptoclastic (destructive) signalling molecules consist of inflammatory pathway super-regulator NFkB, fungi (moulds), pathogenic bacteria, trans-fats and AGEs and the synaptoblastic inducing molecules of omega-3 fats, vitamin C, CoQ10 and various phytonutrients..

Inflammation is an inevitable result of certain diets and leaky gut (combined with certain genetic predispositions) which translates to leaky brain too (remember the blood brain barrier is like the gut barrier). A high sugar and processed carb diet actually shrinks your brain! When you cut out the carbs, and add good fats (nuts, olive oil) to your diet then you can do much to prevent the development of AD. You are changing your brain chemistry by the chronic consumption of a high carbohydrate diet![105] Equally you can reverse it with a high fat/moderate protein/low processed-carbs diet.

Thyroid Function and Dementia

There is a particular association of low thyroid function or hypothyroidism and memory loss related to dementia: This is caused by low thyroxine (T3 – the main thyroid hormone), high reverse T3 (rT3 – an altered molecule which does not fit the receptor properly) and elevation of the inflammatory markers (cytokines) **tumour necrosis factor alpha** (**TNF-α** or cachexin) and **interleukin 6** (**IL-6**).[106] Cytokines like these are the language of the immune system and their balance is often very significant tending towards either inflammatory or anti-inflammatory signalling.

The data is conflicting however, as studies concentrate on populations not individuals and we know that thyroid function has huge individual variation. What may be normal for one person may too low or high for another. That's why population ranges can be both confusing and unhelpful when determining how much thyroxine a person needs. Much better is to check temperature and how the patient *feels*; they will usually feel terrible without enough T3. Low thyroid function is a problem in many diseases not just dementia but particularly breast cancer, so it makes sense to find out your levels if you are concerned. It is not just a matter of increasing iodine intake, although this may be warranted. The solution is more general: reduce oxidative stress and raise mitochondrial function. As we have already discussed in Chapters 2 and 3, the thyroid concentrates toxins and so will struggle if the body is toxic.

Preventative Dementia Treatments

Quite apart from eating good food, getting better sleep, dealing with your stress/unresolved emotions, there are various specific interventions that are showing huge promise.

Vitamin D and Alzheimer's

"During the last 25 years, vitamin D has emerged as a serious candidate in nervous system development and function and a therapeutic tool in a number of neurological pathologies."[107] It is especially powerful against neurodegenerative diseases such as Alzheimer's Disease (AD) and Parkinson's (PD)[i]. Low vitamin D is highly correlated with cognitive decline causing doubling in the risk of AD[108] and non-Alzheimer's dementia[109], particularly in ethnic minorities.[110] It doesn't stop there; vitamin D isn't only promising as an agent of risk reduction but also as a treatment that can reverse neurodegenerative decline.

"Supplementation with vitamin D has such potent benefits for the brain because the brain relies on vitamin D receptors for protection against a variety of destructive processes. Vitamin D has been shown to have a critical role in nerve cell growth and differentiation, nerve transmission, and the "plasticity" of connections that's so essential for normal learning and memory[111]. Without adequate vitamin D, all of those functions suffer, and some fail.[112]

---

[i] It reduces the severity of Parkinson's

141

Turmeric

Turmeric has been shown to profoundly alter the development of the disease for instance, reversing some symptoms to the point that patients begin to recognise their family again after a year of taking it. However, you won't see turmeric therapy being offered in your GP clinic anytime soon; the trials are simply not supported as they are non-patentable being foods and therefore no pharmaceutical companies will fund the very expensive trials. But read the literature and make up your own mind.[113]

Coconut Oil and the Ketogenic Diet

If you can lower insulin resistance by reducing carb intake and increasing good fat in your diet to promote ketogenesis, then you can reduce inflammation. Coconut oil is one method of doing this – it contains a high proportion (60 – 65%) of a type of saturated fat called **Medium-Chain-Triglycerides** (**MCTs**– sometimes also called medium chain fatty acids or MCFAs) which are highly neuro-protective. There are also commercially branded products which have been distilled to increase the amount of these fats – called MCT Oil, etc. Daily ingestion of a tablespoon (working up to this amount over several weeks and giving digestive support if necessary) has been shown to reduce cognitive symptoms by a significant amount[114].

Brain Training - New learning

There has been recent interest in the idea of keeping the brain active in order to prevent deterioration. The idea that the brain is fixed is now defunct –we know from an understanding of neuroplasticity that the brain can grow its neuronal connections *according to need* i.e. 'use it or lose it'. But according to expert neuroscientist Lisa Genova, it is not just about doing some crosswords! These activities are, in fact, just remembering what you *already know* and therefore do not recruit new circuits in the brain (a feature which is essential for neuroplasticity). If we understand that it is the *recruitment of new pathways* that is important to increase neuroplasticity, then learning a new skill or language would be better.

These new skills must involve sight, sound and emotions in order to build new neuronal connections – a factor that is essential in the building of what she calls 'cognitive reserve'. We normally lose neurons as we age, but if we've built up a reserve of extra neurons from new meaning–rich learning during our active years, then this acts as a buffer to give us backup to the inevitable loss later on. So learning a new skill (a language, craft or musical skill like singing) is important in middle age as a preventative factor. But it is not too late to do something even if you are showing signs of some memory loss.

The best interventions combine all of these lifestyle interventions into one programme: the Bredesen protocol in the US and the FINGER study in Sweden are two such programmes showing huge promise in reversing cognitive decline and in prevention. And small changes reap big rewards. According to the study lead author: "Postponing of the onset of Alzheimer's disease by 5 years has been estimated to decrease its prevalence by up to 50% in 50 years[115]" so prevention has to be the focus of our attention now rather than the development of a new 'wonder drug'. These have been spectacularly unsuccessful so far because they are based on an out of date model of the body.

Leading functional medical doctor Raphael Kellman has said: "there is no human being that cannot be helped whatever stage of disease; they may not regain their memory, but the progress can be arrested and with the help of education they can be given back some functions". This makes sense to me. If, as we now know, AD begins early in middle age as a whole body response to poor sugar metabolism or toxicity with concomitant changes in mitochondrial function, then we can surmise it should be reversible to some degree, depending on what stage we are at and what interventions we use.

There is certainly hope to be had and many alternatives to the current pharmacological route which does little to arrest the disease and costs Western nations billions they can ill afford.

Age-related Macular Degeneration - AMD

This common condition is the "leading cause of blindness in the elderly worldwide" and is characterised by loss of sight in the centre of vision. It is seen mostly in people over 50 hence the name **age-related macular degeneration (AMD)**. However, as I have already been at pains to express, it has nothing to do with normal ageing but more to poor anti-oxidant status and 'bad' light (too much UVB) which damages the central part of the retina (the **macula**). There are two types: wet (a build-up of blood vessels in the macula) and dry (slow degeneration of the macula). It is a condition for which western medicine has limited treatments although wet is treated better than dry[116].

There are huge parallels with Alzheimer's as it is also characterized by the formation of glycated proteins, inflammatory mediators and AGEs in pockets called **drusen** in the macula. The presence of drusen characterise the disease much like amyloid protein does in AD.

Considerable attention is now being focused on nutritional treatments as conventional medical treatments are usually aimed at keeping the sight loss stable only after it has already begun.[117]

CFS/ME

CFS/ME is not normally considered a disease of ageing or neurodegenerative, but as its primary symptoms – brain fog and fatigue - are symptoms of neuro-inflammation, I want to tackle it briefly here (for more detailed information please refer to my first book). Long considered a mystery disease by conventional medicine, it is now becoming clear it is a *functional metabolic condition* with whole body systemic effects. The systems of the body begin to close down and function becomes minimal –just enough to keep the person alive but with no quality of life whatsoever.

For a long time this was considered to be a psychiatric disorder 'made up' by the person for reasons unknown. However, thankfully for the millions of sufferers, recent research is showing real, measurable cellular changes which may account for the myriad symptoms. According to pre-eminent mitochondrial researcher' Robert Naviaux[118], this downshift is a function of the Cell Danger Response (CDR) as already discussed which causes mitochondria to:

1. shift from efficient ATP/ADP energy metabolism to inefficient cytosol (cellular fluid) production outside
2. increase mitochondrial **autophagy** (break up and destruction)
3. change their DNA methylation and histone modification to up-regulate pathogenenic (disease-causing) gene expression[i]
4. warn neighbouring cells and effector cells with release of extracellular nucleotides, peroxide, eicosanoids and cytokines, etc

---

[i]For instance, pathogenic bacteria methylate (add methyl groups to) mercury in your gut causing all sorts of problems.

It is meant to be short-term but, if it persists, the whole body metabolism is disturbed. Further problems occur because according to researchers::

"when the danger is past and cellular function is restored, a metabolic memory is stored in a way similar to the way the brain stores memories, in the form of durable changes in mitochondrial biomass and cellular protein, lipid and other macromolecule content (metabolomics[i]), cell structure and gene expression via somatic (body-based) epigenetic modifications. This cellular memory is also called **mitocellular hormesis**[119] and is under the control of ancient parts of the brain (the brainstem) which ... may explain the psychological effects".[120]

The cell responds by closing down to minimise wastage of resources and protect its molecular machinery. Far from being just collateral damage,

"the fatigue in ME/CFS is due to an active and purposeful inhibition of mitochondria. The mitochondria are not broken – they're throttled back to a low idle. In the face of danger, they shut down and export ATP outside the cell to warn other cells that danger is present. The latest research concludes that "genes, environment and timing all conspire to create ME/CFS"[121]

And of all the exposures, it seems that adverse childhood events (ACE's) are the most significant cause leading to this condition. They cause an altered stress response via the HPA axis that sets the stage for problems years later. If the body considers itself on high alert the whole time because of unresolved emotional events in childhood[ii], then all the body's systems are affected.[122] Fibromyalgia, a similar condition but with pain as its main symptom, has recently been redefined as needing to have childhood trauma in the patient's history to be properly considered Fibro[iii].

So, in effect CFS/ME/Fibro are both 'warning sign' diseases of accelerated ageing and cellular shutdown. It IS reversible despite what modern medicine and the benefits system encourages you to believe, but it takes a systems (functional) medicine approach to deal with all the systems that are dysfunctional. I refer you to my first book for more info on this condition and the various programmes that aim to reverse it[iv].

---

[i]Metabolomics (study of cell's metabolites) as a 'disease signature' is a huge area of interest at the moment, especially with respect to chronic disease states like CFS/ME
[ii] Traumatic emotional events are dealt with in the same part of the brain that deals with survival – the limbic system and may be interpreted by the brain as an ongoing threat
[iii] See the work of David Brady
[iv]There are various options: The Chrysalis Effect, Optimum Health Clinic, Gupta programme, Irene Lyons, and Ari Whitten's programmes amongst many others.

Depression and Anxiety

There is a new model of depression which links it to cellular health rather than a deficiency of neurotransmitters per se. Brain cells take up a lot of our energy (around 30% of our total output - and much more in children) because brain cells (neurons) are very densely populated with mitochondria (energy factories of the cell). We know that mood is largely governed by a careful balance of neurotransmitters and connectivity between brain regions, in particular the frontal lobes which transmit calming messages of safety and judgment of risk. But when the neuro-inflammation is present[i], inflammatory cytokines are produced which suppress the frontal lobes. This lack of activity means that mood regulation fails to occur and depression is inevitable. Thus it is not the chemical imbalance (lack of serotonin) as the current medical model would have you believe. The gut/brain/skin axis has been known about for over 100 years but the knowledge has been suppressed in favour of the chemical imbalance theory which sells antidepressant drugs. Suffice to say once neuro-inflammation has started it signals to the cells the Cell Danger Response and an immune response is initiated which becomes difficult to dampen – it becomes chronic and stuck in the energy conserving mode of parasympathetically induced freeze.

Chronic neuro-inflammation, which is what depression is, actually decreases the firing rate of neurons in your brain so can give concomitant symptoms of brain fog, slow reflexes and poor recall. None of these symptoms are improved by the drugs currently used to treat depression – we need to deal with the gut inflammation first and add in some of the missing amino acids (building blocks of proteins) that are consequently lacking. L-thiamine and tyrosine are two of the most important. For more information on this I refer you to the work of Trudy Scott and her excellent book on treating depression with specific nutrients.[123] There is, of course, my own book, The Scar that Won't Heal, that looked at the other cause of toxic stress.

Multiple Sclerosis

Multiple sclerosis is an auto-immune disease of degradation of the myelin sheath of the nerves which decreases their ability to function and so motor and muscle problems ensue. It is likely an extreme effect of long term stress

---

[i] because of systemic inflammation of the gut – remember the gut and brain are very similar tissues and share a blood supply i.e. leaky gut = leaky brain

and chronic deficiency and toxicity. One of the highest correlations is a lack of vitamin D in the body.

MS is a disease that has long mystified medics- with its classic remission and relapses, it seems to play itself out in odd ways. However with a functional medicine hat on we see that in fact it makes perfect sense that when detoxification is working, remission is possible, but with a high toxic burden relapse is inevitable. We need to support the body systems that promote detoxification and reduce the toxic burden.

Vitamin D3

We've talked about the roles of vitamin D extensively in the previous chapter but just to note recent research "provides significant evidence that vitamin D is also involved in the regeneration of myelin[124]. And prevalence of the disease is linked with lower vitamin D levels. Although not enough to conclude lack of vitamin D *causes* MS, this indicates it is *associated* with it in significant ways. Certainly optimizing your vitamin D levels to at least 75ng/ml (much higher than the levels recommended currently in government RDAs) is going to be important. But this is not enough. There are other nutrients that need to be supplied in optimal doses in order for the neurons to work well.

Vitamin K2

New information is coming to light that MS may be linked to a lack of vitamin K as well as D3 (they are linked as D3 is needed to activate K2). It has been noted that people with MS even have ¼ of the K2 levels of non-MS patients. K2 inhibits inflammation and the accumulation of reactive oxygen species (ROS) and thus may be a future treatment for Multiple Sclerosis (MS) and even Parkinson's.

Mitochondrial Treatments for MS

Remember, these neuro-degenerative diseases have common features of mitochondrial dysfunction so what works for neuro-degeneration generally will work for MS and PD. Terry Wahls healed herself of MS using nutrition and now talks about this[125]. She maintains omega-3 fatty acids (from seed oils, fish and grass-fed meat), B vitamins, iodine, and antioxidants like co-enzyme Q10, Alpha lipoic acid (ALA) and L-carnitine. Adaptogenic[i] herbs like ginseng, ashwaganda and rhodiola have been shown to be helpful in that they reduce cortisol levels (a potent driver of inflammation when chronic). Finally MCT oil (sometimes referred to as 'brain-octane' oil and low dose Naltrexone can all be helpful. But mainly, your diet needs to be adjusted to one of high amounts (3 cups a day) of leafy greens – particularly the cabbage and onion families[i] because of the high sulphur. Expect it to take 1 – 2 years to normalize but you will notice improvements within a month or so.

Parkinson's Disease

Parkinson's Disease (PD) is a progressive neurodegenerative disease like Alzheimer's but receives less funding or general awareness affecting 1 in every 37 people. According to a recent report, its prevalence and incidence is likely to double by 2065[126] so it is not something that we can ignore.

It has long been known that PD is a problem of brain damage to an area called the **substantia nigra (SN)** which is involved with control of movement. The three diagnostic symptoms are:

1. Shaking – (a pill-rolling movement of the hand)
2. Stiffness of limbs
3. Slowed or poor motor control - bradykinesia

Parkinson's, like Alzheimer's, has always been considered a problem of the brain with a loss of dopamine production by the SN leading to a type of palsy (indeed Dr Parkinson, who first identified it, called it the 'shaking palsy'). The disease has since come to bear his name. But even now expert researchers and clinicians are stumped as to how to cure it. Their best treatment is administering L-dopa, together with artificial agonists (keys in the receptor lock) which have considerable side effects and thus not well tolerated by many people. It is not well treated conventionally therefore.

Researchers know that the problem of protein aggregation in the neurons (similar to Alzheimer's but a different protein[ii]) is the brain's response to inflammation propagated by the gradual down-regulation of mitochondria. Neurons are very energy hungry as we've seen and every time movement is required a huge number are recruited to control the movement which

---

[i] Means they adapt the system up or down whatever is needed. No drug does this.
[i] Kale, cabbage, broccoli, spring greens, onions, leeks, garlic and shallots
[ii] misfolded alpha-synuclein into intracellular aggregates called Lewy Bodies

involves many different brain areas besides the SN. It is just that the SN has the most obvious changes (it is called the substantia nigra or 'black substance' in Latin because it looks black under the microscope.

It has been observed that many mitochondria in the SN die without replacement leading to loss of dopamine release (in this case) leading to a lack of control of movement. Cell biologists have identified a crucial protein, which they have dubbed 'parkin', which promotes fusion and motility (both essentials to good neuronal function). Parkin is a protein often mutated in PD. It seems that lack of parkin causes an imbalance to the fusion/fission cycle with more fission and thus less ATP (energy currency). The mutation may be induced by specific pesticides[127] or drugs[i]. We have already noted that PD is more common in farm workers and less so in smokers (an inverse correlation strangely)[128] but there may also be a link with glutathione metabolism via the GST gene SNiP. People vary in the genetic mutations they inherit and GST is one gene that has a common variance – some people inherit a version that is less efficient at recycling glutathione, one of the most powerful antioxidants in the body.

However, not being aware that mitos talk to your gut flora (being bacterial in origin) and that the gut and the brain are embryologically the same tissue, has hindered understanding up to now. It is plain that inflammation begins in the gut and treatment of dysbiosis (unbalanced gut flora) helps inhibit inflammation and oxidative stress and may be a future treatment for PD

Similarly to what we saw with Alzheimer's and MS, Vitamin D can benefit people with Parkinson's disease as well. In humans, it's already known that vitamin D supplementation reduces falls and improves balance in healthy older adults - two problems often faced by patients with Parkinson's. "A randomized, placebo-controlled clinical trial has shown that 1,200 IU/day of vitamin D3 prevents deterioration in Parkinson's disease patients over a 12-month period. Intriguingly, this effect depended on the patients' type of vitamin D receptors in brain tissue." [52]

---

[i] A batch of heroin laced with a substance called MPTP was blamed for an outbreak of Parkinsonian symptoms in young men in California in the 1980's. But it led to many of the understandings we have now or what goes wrong in this disease.

Chapter 8: Cancer - A Metabolic Adaptation

Cancer is such a politicised arena and cultural taboo that it makes it hard to discuss rationally. I covered some of the politics of current health funding and research in my last book The World Within so I don't aim to repeat that here. The important point to note is that the dominant theory of cancer initiation has been one of accumulating genetic damage causing the uncontrolled proliferation of cells. Whilst this is basically correct it is not a random act by a bewildered, un-co-ordinated cell. The truth is more that it is, in fact, *a highly co-ordinated response to perceived environmental threat and toxicity* with a survival response. We will discuss how the cell responds to such threat later on but first I need to introduce the old and new paradigms.

The Cancer Conundrum

It seems not a week goes by without some new 'cancer breakthrough' is announced. Currently the best new conventional approach showing promise is immunotherapy, which, although still not the magic bullet everyone is seeking[129], seems to be more targeted than the conventional approaches of radiation, surgery and chemotherapy (what I think of as 'slash and burn' – a therapy largely unchanged in 100 years!). However, all of these treatments, old and new are based on the view of cancer as a disease of rogue cells randomly replicating 'out of control' to form a tumour due to faulty genetic instructions. I remember learning this model with its four stages (stages I through to IV) and feeling very depressed, as it seemed both random and somewhat inevitable (1 in 2 men and 1 in 3 women at the moment are predicted to contract some form of cancer in their lifetime). But what if these theories are based on a faulty understanding of cancer? Could that not explain why, despite years of

---

Compared to 1 in 8000 in 1900. Our genetics have not changed that rapidly but our environment has.

151

increasing research spending, we seem to be no nearer the cure for cancer? Clearly we are not winning the 'war on cancer[i]' as rates rise inexorably.

Conventional Cancer Treatment

Current treatments focus mostly on destroying the errant cells i.e. the tumour, which is regarded as the problem (rather than the result of the problem). In order to do this modern medicine has 3 approaches; removal (surgery), burning (radiation) and killing cancer cells (chemotherapy). Most chemotherapy drugs were derived from pesticides and are very powerful immune modulators via their interaction with the gut microbiome[130]. A powerful inflammatory response from the microbiome is triggered to enhance immunity to attack cancer cells. But it is a very blunt instrument and kills *all* rapidly dividing cells including hair and gut lining with disastrous results. Chemo is one of the few treatments that could be said to be worse than the disease itself. It causes tremendous suffering, but is sometimes successful for people whose immune systems are robust enough. However there are many for whom it only works temporarily and then the cancer 'comes back'[ii] even more vigorously than before. Yes people live longer with some cancers, and some do indeed get remission. But overall, cancer rates are rising and success rates (defined as cancer free for 5 years – note *only* 5 years) are not much different now from the 1950's. Despite what the media trumpets, we are not really making much headway in curing cancer this way.

This idea that we can 'get all the cancer' is a misunderstanding of what cancer is and does. It is not like an infection as that terminology would seem to imply[iii]. It can't 'come back' in that way. It is an internal epigenetic switch that gets turned on by a toxic cellular environment not an external threat. If nothing in the lifestyle of that person has changed then all the conditions for the systemic development of cancer are still present and the same dysfunction is likely therefore. It may develop in a different part of the body (the weakest link in the chain at the time). But it is not a vicious predator waiting to strike but a defence mechanism of the body to try to

---

[i] As declared by the American government in 1971
[ii] You often read about such cases in news and social media. Phrases like 'they didn't get it all' or 'it came back worse than ever' are misleading – they misunderstand that cancer is not the tumour itself– but a process throughout the body – the tumour is the most obvious sign (usually in the weakest spot) but it is not the only problem – cancer is systemic.
[iii] Cancer is not in fact a disease but a survival mechanism to extreme cellular toxicity

enable it to survive! This is a vastly different understanding that may at first sound difficult to swallow as it so contradicts the conventional understanding. Let me explain further.

Cancer cells preferentially use glycolysis (energy production within the cell matrix –see Chapter 2) so needs vast amounts of glucose (hence the name glyco- (sugar) lysis (breakup). When blood glucose runs out, the body is forced to use up its reserves of fat stores to convert into glucose – hence huge weight loss is often a feature of cancer (**cachexia**). In a mistaken attempt to build the patient up again, sufferers are often recommended to eat carb- rich and sugar-filled foods. This is a terrible idea, as it simply perpetuates the imbalance – much better would be high fat, low carb (**ketogenic**) diet, high in essential fats like flax oil, avocados, nuts and seeds plus high polyphenols (plant chemicals containing anti-oxidants) from coloured vegetables and green tea, etc. For full details see one of the many excellent research-supported books on the subject.[131,132]

There is so much you can do to help yourself and those you love with this disease. Don't assume the victim role and take back control – even something as simple as fasting the day before chemo (allowing 36 hours before your chemo) will make a huge difference to how you feel afterwards. There is less nausea, less hair loss and general malaise[i]. Another simple recommendation is to give high dose broad-spectrum probiotics or fermented foods to people undergoing chemotherapy. It helps to restore the microbiome which is devastated by the chemo. When the gut flora is re-established, it begins to talk to the immune system again and produces compounds to heal the gut wall. Sadly this is seldom done in current medical practice, with the result of a great deal of suffering.

A New Theory of Cancer

The conventional theory of cancer as taught in medical schools are that cancer is a result of injury to the genes such that cells start to behave as single cells, not part of an organism. They have forgotten they belong to a large organism. The cell becomes so damaged, it cannot be repaired. Thus the only thing left for it to do is to start dividing. This rapid cell division is the essential cell biology of cancer, as each generation passes on this poor

---

[i] As described by Dr Nasha Winters in her online presentation about Cancer as a metabolic disease, referencing the work of Dr Valter Longo – see his book The Longevity Diet.

repair to their daughter genes so that growth is then exponential (the basis of the tumour - a cluster of large, overgrowing cells). But there are several holes in the theory that are unexplained. What causes the cells to go rogue? With all that we now about how tightly co-ordinated cellular life is and epigenetic variation, it seems insufficient explanation to say that random mutation is the cause, based on your genetic endowment and bad luck. This so-called **Somatic Mutation Theory (SMT)** is inadequate at least and downright wrong at best. We need to look at other competing theories to see if they explain things a bit more robustly.

Over the history of cancer research there have developed two basic (and slightly competing) theories of cancer initiation: *genetic* (random mutation) versus *mitochondrial* (co-ordinated metabolic). No prizes for guessing which view I favour. It simply makes no sense that an intelligent, co-ordinated system like the body would destroy itself randomly (the same is also true of auto-immune conditions of course). A great deal of research effort has gone into looking at the minutiae of cellular changes to the genome in the effort to find the molecular 'switch' so we can turn it off. Like most of these reductionist genetic approaches seeking to find the 'cure for x', it is doomed to failure.[i] The secret is surely the **terrain**, or extra-cellular space – something that is seldom looked at by cancer researchers.

It is known that cancer cells develop hyper-resistance to normal checks and balances, adopting the survival strategy of a single-celled organism – this is one of the 'hallmarks of cancer'[133][ii] and is termed the **'cancer paradox'**. Why would this be? It is not simply a genetic malfunction as the SMT would have it. There are numerous holes in this idea; for instance it has been noted that if you transfer the nuclei from cancerous cells and put them into non-cancerous cells, the cells do not become cancerous (which would be expected if cancer was purely genetic – remember the cell's genes (DNA – including the cancer switching genes) are mostly in the nucleus. However, if you transfer the **cytoplasm** (cell fluid) from cancerous to non-cancerous cells, the adoptive cells become cancerous[134]. Clearly there is something in

---

[i] There are a few more truly genetic cancers that afflict children and young adults but most (up to 75%) are lifestyle diseases. So looking for the one gene is likely to fail.

[ii] The full list described by Hanahan and Weinberg is: Cancer cells 1) stimulate their own growth (2) resist growth inhibitory signals (3) resist programmed cell death (**apoptosis**); (4) multiply indefinitely (5) stimulate the growth of blood vessels to supply nutrients o tumours (**angiogenesis**); (6) invade local tissue and spread to distant sites (**metastasis**). (7) have abnormal metabolic pathways (8) evade the immune system

the cytoplasm that is signalling a cancerous message – maybe high amounts of cellular debris/acidity or hypoxia. Something that is picked up by the cellular sensing mechanism as a Cell Danger Response to down-regulate metabolism, switching it to low energy fermentation (glycolysis). This cellular sensing mechanism has subsequently been identified as the mitochondria - mitochondrial DNA (mtDNA) and its products. Mitochondria, therefore, are at the heart of cancer too.

Mitochondria and Cancer

We now know that: "mtDNA can be transferred horizontally from host cells to tumour cells in the microenvironment"[135]. In other words, mtDNA transfers from the mitochondria of non-cancerous and cancerous cells swapping information and changing the signalling towards one or the other *dependent on the environment*. Remember, "replication of mtDNA is *not* subject to the normal cell cycle of division and replication (unlike the nuclear DNA) and may be performed many times without the checks and balances of that process. This leads to generation of mtDNA mutations by replication errors in addition to ones due to accumulated damage."[136] DNA is very liable to damage by free radicals (ROS) produced by normal metabolism (in the ETC) and that is why mtDNA so is vulnerable as it lies outside the nucleus and is not protected. Thus genetics are involved, but they are not solely nuclear DNA determined – these mutations are *downstream* from the initiating events, hence our failure to reverse cancer by targeting such nuclear mutations.

This is what led innovative cancer researchers Seyfried and D'Agostino to the idea that cancer is a *mitochondrial, metabolic response to threat*, and mitochondrial signalling of the cell danger response has a large part to play. This theory is not a new one; it was being developed as early as the 1950's by a eminent researcher called Otto Warburg whose theories were initially welcomed and then largely ignored with the advent of the Human Genome Project and the Big Pharma-driven push to finding the 'gene for everything'. In particular, the Cancer Genome Atlas, begun in 2006, aimed to find the genetic signature for cancerous cells and largely failed due to inconsistencies in the data (we now know this is due to different epigenetic expressions of the nuclear DNA). This research initiative has largely failed to provide any significant breakthroughs in magic bullet therapies. For more information I refer you to two excellent books on the subject[137,138]

Warburg Hypothesis – Cancer as a Metabolic Disease

Otto Warburg postulated that cancer is, first and foremost, a *metabolic disease* of hyper-fermentation of glucose (glycolysis) resulting in genetic mutations. Note again that the mutations are downstream of the initiating problem (cause) *not the cause itself.* He first identified that:

"in conditions of poor oxygenation, mitochondria will switch energy production away from the efficient mechanism of oxidative phosphorylation, towards low efficiency glycolysis outside of the mitos. However, this isn't a one-way switch but a highly intelligent response towards survival of the whole. It seems that mitochondria pick up the danger message of threat to the system and shut themselves down in order to protect the cell from damage."

When cells have to divide, as is the case with systemic threat and inflammation, nuclear DNA becomes vulnerable to damage from free radicals (reactive oxygen species – ROS- or 'rust') formed naturally as part of the mitochondrial energy cycle of oxidative phosphorylation (respiration or oxyphos). So energy production has to be intelligently switched to the alternative pathway outside the mitos called glycolysis (fermentation) *to protect the DNA during mitosis* (cell division). This would normally be switched on again when conditions of division have ended. Without the highly information-rich ATP molecules that are produced within the mitos by oxyphos, the cells lose signalling data and fail to regulate their growth. The system becomes dysregulated, toxic and tumours can result. This process of switching to preferential glycolysis is termed the 'Warburg Effect' and is essential to a new understanding of cancer formation.

Table 3: Warburg Effect - Updated

Low oxygen	High oxygen	Moderate but insufficient oxygen
glycolysis (fermentation)	oxidative phosphorylation (respiration)	aerobic glycolysis (elective fermentation)
anaerobic (without oxygen)	aerobic (with oxygen)	aerobic (with oxygen)
low efficiency	high efficiency	low efficiency
in cytosol – cell fluid	within mitochondria	in cytosol – cell fluid
cancer promoting	cancer inhibiting	cancer promoting

However, this idea has been updated even further with the understanding that the cells can in fact *choose* which type of energy production they favour - *even in the presence of oxygen*. It isn't just a mechanistic switch depending on oxygen levels as to whether they go. When they go to the low efficiency glycolytic (sugar-breakdown) route in the presence of oxygen, this is called *aerobic* **glycolysis** and this plays a major role in **carcinogenesis** (cancer initiation) and **tumourigenesis (**tumour growth).

"Understanding the mechanisms involved in the metabolic switch between oxidative phosphorylation and aerobic glycolysis may therefore be important for the development of potential preventive and therapeutic interventions."[139]

As this process continues, certain metabolites (chemical products of metabolism) leak out from the mitos to the nucleus and *deactivate* suppressors of **oncogenes** (cancer promoting genes). In other words they switch off the brake and cells can suddenly start proliferating madly – attracting a greater blood supply by the development of new blood vessels (**angiogenesis)** and lymph vessels (lymphangiogenesis)[i]. The cells lose their central co-ordination and start to behave as if they were individual cells as a survival strategy! Thus in this new updated understanding somatic mutations are epiphenomena (later events occurring after carcinogenesis is already underway). This would explain why we have had such little luck with most of the research effort directed at changing the genetics of cancer. It is too far downstream - akin to 'closing the stable door after the horse has bolted', as they say!

Alterations to Cellular Function

Cancer cells not only have altered metabolism of their mitochondria as we have seen, but they accumulate more damaged mitochondria due to a loss of normal recycling of those damaged cells by **apoptosis** (programmed cell suicide) and **autophagy** (mitochondrial self-destruction/recycling). Mitochondria are acutely tuned to their environment. If they detect an unsatisfactory one, they will signal their own destruction - a normal part of keeping the cell healthy. Remember when looking at neuro-degenerative disease in the last Chapter it was the balance of mitochondrial fission and fusion that dictated the efficiency of mitochondria. Well in cancer cells we actually want to *enhance* destruction of the aberrant cells i.e. fission and

---

[i] I apologise there are so many technical words in the field of cancer research!

apoptosis. This is a new target for intervention along with the molecular switching between mechanisms as detailed above.

In natural medicine there are always multiple ways of achieving the desired result – as well as multiple ways in which one can develop a disease. It is not simply a 'one size fits all approach'. Another potential intervention currently under investigation is manipulating the pH (acidity) of the cell environment.

Cell pH

The cell pH describes the acidity levels inside the cell; a higher pH is alkaline (above pH7) and a lower number (below 7) indicates acidic. It has been posited by some in the alternative health community that the main difference between cancer promotion and inhibition is the pH of blood. But this is disputed by the official Cancer Research bodies[i] and with good reason. Blood pH is tightly controlled by mechanisms that involve calcium uptake or deposition. If your blood pH changed by even 0.5 on the pH scale you would be in serious trouble!

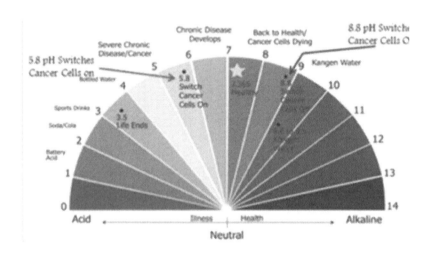

Figure 49: pH and Cancer

---

[i] See Cancer Research UK '10 Myths of Cancer'. Some are accurate but not all. Lemons for instance do require an alkaline response from the body so are alkalizing.

How about the pH of the intra-cellular environment of the cell? Could that have anything to do with cancer promotion or initiation? This **intra-cellular pH** varies but is normally controlled to within 7.2 – 7.4 (slightly alkaline) to maintain normal metabolism, despite what is happening outside the cell from various external modifications. Factors such as type of food (meat, eggs and dairy products tend to be acidifying to the external cell environment whereas vegetables are alkalising), exercise (moderate exercise is generally alkalizing, stress levels (high stress is acidifying), etc. What has all this got to do with cancer? Quite a lot it seems.

The cell maintains its intracellular pH relative to the extracellular environment (**pH gradient**) by means of its **proton pumps** which straddle the membrane and continually pump out protons (H^+ ions)[i]. It has been noticed that cancer cells possess a *reversed* pH gradient i.e. a higher internal (more alkaline) pH and a lower external pH than normal cells[ii] – called 'intracellular alkalinization'[140]. Recently it has been proposed by Calderon that "even in the presence of adequate oxygen levels, the intracellular pH may play a key role in determining the way cells obtain energy; an alkaline internal pH driving aerobic glycolysis (cancer fermentation) and an acidic pH driving oxidative phosphorylation (normal respiration)"[16]. As this process continues, according to Seyfried it becomes self-perpetuating by promoting:

"a protracted shift from respiration (oxyphos) to fermentation (glycolysis) that will acidify and destabilize the tissue microenvironment. Microenvironment acidification enhances angiogenesis and facilitates the path to tumourigenesis" [116,131]

This may indeed be the 'unifying theory' that brings together all cancers as having this one electrochemical driving force common to all. This flies in the face of current medical dogma that cancers are hundreds of different diseases all requiring novel independent treatments depending on the tumour site. I have always been suspicious of this theory which I hear touted frequently in the media whenever a medical 'expert' is called in to explain the latest new treatment, but I now know that the research simply doesn't support it.

---

[i] The more protons (H^+) it pumps out the higher the acidity levels outside the cell and the lower (higher pH) inside the cell. This is a cancer promoting situation.
[ii] Tumour cells have internal pHi values of 7.12–7.7 versus 6.99–7.05 in normal cells while producing acidic cytosolic pHe values of 6.2–6.9 versus 7.3–7.4 in normal cells. This creates a reversed pH gradient across the cell membrane which drives cancer.

Oxygen deprivation may be the main initiating factor but after that pH may play a supporting role driving tumourigenesis. In simple terms a higher internal pH (more alkaline cell) drives the mechanisms that switch the cell to a cancerous energy metabolism. The lower pH externally is also important as "adaptations to this highly acidic microenvironment are critical steps in transition from an avascular pre-invasive tumour to a malignant invasive carcinoma[141]". So an acidic external environment to the cell may not just trigger cancer but help it develop via angiogenesis (the growth of new blood vessels to support the tumour growth).

So, how do we create an alkaline external cell environment of the body ('alkalosis')? We can do this by ingesting alkaline forming foods (mainly green vegetables – juiced ideally if the digestion is poor. Remember:

"the increased intracellular alkalosis is a strong mitogenic signal, which bypasses most inhibitory signals. Concomitant correction of this alkalosis may be a very effective treatment in case of mitochondrial failure".[142]

Here is where the information on sites such as Cancer Research UK or similar industry-fed charities is wrong. It says and I quote: "there's no good evidence to prove that diet can manipulate whole body pH, *or that it has an impact on cancer*"[143] (my italics). Now I can't comment on 'whole body pH' whatever that means (extracellular fluid? blood?) but there is a whole raft of evidence that diet very effectively manipulates cancer development and risk. I refer you to the many excellent books on the subject such as those by Dr Servan-Schreiber and Richard Beliveau which are fully referenced[144,145]. These are not 'quacks' or alternative health gurus but highly respected researchers and cancer experts. To say diet has no impact on cancer is willfully (and industry-sponsored) misinformation. It is tantamount to malpractice when it comes from the mouths of oncologists. But sadly that is the case.[i]

Cell Signalling Changes

Remember the cell is under tight control of its reproductive and proliferative capacities. But something happens when cells turn cancerous.

---

[i] I have a colleague who died a few months after being told by his oncologist to eat cakes and anything sugary to build himself up in the recovery period after radiation treatment for stomach cancer. I was aghast but was unable to persuade him this was wrong advice.

"While the growth and survival of normal cells are under partial control from growth factors and hormones, alterations in signalling pathways, resulting from mutations and/or epigenetic changes, renders cells resistant and independent of these pathways. Such changes promote survival and growth both by constitutively stimulating pathways that favor proliferation, and by inhibiting and/or overriding apoptotic pathways. Initially, altered signalling pathways, as well as changes in the metabolomics profile (products of metabolism), epigenetically modify the patterns of gene expression in the cell, and as such are therapeutically reversible"[146]

Note that word in the last line: *reversible*. Let's now look at cellular inputs that we've already introduced but with a specific lens of cancer and ways to intervene in cancer.

Kinase Network and Nutrients

In Chapter 2 we looked at the kinase network as a way that the external environment of the cell triggers a cascade of reactions inside the cell to enact a response. It is one of the 'relays' of the cell which act to turn on the **natural killer (NK)** cells of the cell-mediated immune system.

Certain natural nutrients induce the kinase network to promote more NK cells. **Sulphoraphane** (an organo-sulphur compound found in broccoli and sprouts) is one of the most potent and therefore a fantastic anti-cancer compound alongside **curcumin**, resveratrol (in red wine & grapes), indole-3-carbinol (I-3C) & brassinin (in brassicas), epigallocatechin-3-gallate (E-3-G in green tea), genistein, ellagitannins, lycopene (in tomatoes) and quercetin). Some of them we've met before in the Chapter where I introduced you to phyto-nutrients. They have all been found to inhibit pathways contributing to proliferation (uncontrolled cell growth): NFkB, phosphoinositide-3 kinase, insulin growth factor- receptor 1 (IGF-R1), cell cycle-associated proteins, as well as androgen and oestrogen receptor signalling. Notice that last one – remembering that many forms of breast cancer are hormone (particularly oestrogen) positive cancers.

Telomerase and Cancer

One of the messages passed on to the cell is to increase telomere length – by increasing telomerase enzyme activity which repairs telomeres. Remember telomeres control cell senescence (ageing and replacement) and in a healthy cell telomerase is necessary to regulate DNA stability during cell division. But when a cell acquires genetic damage, the telomerase acts to prevent the cells from dying and provide what scientists term 'replicative immortality'[147] i.e. they won't stop dividing. Thus telomere length and telomerase activity are crucial for cancer initiation and the survival of tumours. This doesn't mean telomerase is either good or bad, per se, but that proper regulation has been lost.

Anything that helps us re-regulate cell division and telomere length encourages the cells with genetic damage to be recognised and thus destroyed. The muco-polysaccharides of certain mushrooms like Rieshi, Shitake, etc. are able to do this, hence increasing cell signalling to stop producing cancers. Medicinal mushrooms like this are a vastly under-used intervention which many oncologists would do well to recommend to their patients and preventative charities to their public as the NIH National Cancer Institute in the US have in fact done. They say:

"medicinal mushrooms have been used for hundreds of years, mainly in Asian countries, for treatment of infections. More recently, they have also been used in the treatment of pulmonary diseases and cancer. Medicinal mushrooms have been approved adjuncts to standard cancer treatments in Japan and China for more than 30 years and have an extensive clinical history of safe use as single agents or combined with radiation therapy or chemotherapy mediated through the mushroom's stimulation of innate immune cells, such as monocytes, natural killer cells, and dendritic cells."[148]

It's a startlingly different approach to that of our biggest and richest UK Cancer charity Cancer Research. That's why I won't take part or sponsor a charity run for them or take part in their 'let's beat cancer' charade.

Hypoxia Inducible Factors

We've already considered how a lack of oxygen (**hypoxia)** can switch on tumourigenesis (the development of tumours). We have already described that uncontrolled cellular proliferation is at the heart of the tumour. There is a lack of oxygen in the centre of this rapidly dividing mass, due to natural limitations in the ability of oxygen to diffuse from too distant blood vessels The tumour can only grow blood vessels (angiogenesis) to a certain limit known as 'incomplete vascularisation'. "Tumour cells are thus faced with the challenge of an increased need for nutrients to support the drive for proliferation in the face of a diminished extracellular supply."[149] The cell uses certain cell factors called **hypoxia inducible factors (HIFs)** to increase blood supply. Much has been made of this with certain cancer therapies targeting these HIFs to encourage preventative cell processes[150].

Microbial Correlations

Another contradiction to the notion that cancer is composed of a number of seemingly disparate disease processes i.e. not one disease but many, is the link with microbial DNA. Recently, researchers have found bacterial DNA in tissues with cancer and wondered if the bacterial profile was different to healthy tissue but shared commonalities? They have looked at breast cancer, for instance, and found Sphingomonas bacteria in healthy breast tissue whereas in cancer tissues they found that more methyl bacteria are present. They then asked the question - could the usual processes be being caused by bacteria? i.e. is cancer an infectious disease?. This is probably not the case – it is much more likely that the bacteria are *responding* to the decaying tissue by coming in to help digest it[i]. Support for this theory comes with the fact that aggressive metastatic cancer tissues have no bacteria in them at all – in other words they become more sterile as the cells decay.

There is another theory in fact, and one which I intuitively feel makes sense is that cancer is a response to excess toxicity in the cellular environment that has overwhelmed the body's natural detox mechanisms (lymph, liver, etc). This idea, promulgated by Dr Andreas Moritz, MD in his book[151] is well supported in natural medicine understanding generally where we consider symptoms as the body's attempt to heal itself not the problem. You have to ask the question "what is the purpose of a tumour – and why would the body produce something that threatens its survival? It's much more consistent with the intelligence of the body that it must have an important function. Could switching to aerobic glycolysis help cells (and the tissues and organs they compose) to survive in a low oxygen environment? After all if the essential organs become toxic (especially liver and lymph systems) you will die. Could this be the body's way of ensuring it survives the temporary toxicity (as far as it's concerned)? It is an elegant theory. But modern science is beginning to support this -

Undeniably, the tissues begin to lose connection with other tissues and behave more like solitary cells which divide uncontrollably. This is the basis

---

[i] Indeed this may true with many 'diseases' like Lyme Disease – Borelia species help digest excess sulphur compounds in the blood rather than 'causing the disease.

of metastasis which has conventionally been viewed as the point at which the tumour cells migrate to other parts of the body (metastasise) setting up secondary cancers – this is the invasion (disease) model but it has some problems

Firstly the word metastasis as currently understood occurs is not well understood. It is such a terrifying word and idea. It feels like the body is destroying itself. So much of conventional cancer theory is based on fear messages. Cancer cells may spring up in other places for various reasons due to local injury (egress) – for instance during mammograms small undetected breast tumours may be caused to spread. It seems likely that distribution by the lymph vessels is the likely method of spread being wider than blood vessels and more similar to tissue fluid.[152]. And lymphaniogenesis is widely reported in tumour growth and spread. But again you have to ask why would the body adopt a system that risks its own survival? It can only be because there is a need to do so.

We could look at this another way; if the lymph and detox systems are blocked or insufficient then it makes sense that other cells in different parts of the body would be similarly affected if nothing in the environment changes Overall, cells throughout the body suffer a lack of integrated messages – they have become separated from the 'informational system' of microbiome, mitochondria and immune signalling.

But to summarise, it is unlikely that specific bacterial species *cause* certain cancers (as has been suggested with stomach ulcers and H. pylori for instance). We have to be careful making such sweeping statements as 'correlation is not causation[i]. But we know that the gut is the basis of the innate immune system so it would not be surprising if a dysbiosis (imbalance) in the gut flora was correlated. Time and more research will tell.

Gene Testing

The Somatic Mutation Theory (SMT) of cancer would have it that we need to be genetically tested to determine our risk for cancer. It is the latest in a long line of scientific reductionist theories which ignore all the lifestyle factors. A big push in recent years with the reduction in cost of these

---

[i] Correlations are a scientific distinction that a is found with b – it doesn't mean a causes b – just like smoking and lung disease. Not all smokers get lung disease but it is a very positive correlation - not all lung cancer is caused by smoking. It's complicated!

therapies has been to get your genome sequenced and if it shows a 'cancer gene' (a misunderstanding if ever there was one), then in you are 'doomed' to repeat the intrinsic programming of that gene. This misses out the recent advances in understanding of epigenetics – that no gene is solely responsible for anything – they work in groups which are switched on and off *depending on the cellular environment*. But I digress…

There have been some terrible stories in the press recently about the inaccuracy of some of the algorithms used to provide these 'prognoses'. I would strongly advise only getting yours done from a reputable company and to have a specialist genetic practitioner to go over the results with you. Finding out you have certain 'high risk' genes can be terrible news if you have no understanding of what that means. Let's look at one classic example that has been highly misunderstood.

The BRCA Gene

There has been a lot of focus on the BRCA gene recently after high profile women opted to have their breasts removed when they discovered they had this gene[i]. But be aware – you can be BRCA positive but not cancerous. The standard advice at the moment is if present and there is a history of breast cancer in their families, it is recommended that the woman has her ovaries removed and likely a mastectomy later which supposedly gives a significant breast cancer risk reduction. But not everyone wants to remove a breast or their ovaries and indeed this is licensed mutilation in my opinion. What else can they do? Let's look at other options which are:

1. Improve gut health – reduce gluten and dairy, decrease inflammation and support your flora – reduces the metabolic shift to glycolysis
2. Exercise moderately – this is an epigenetic modifier for an anti-inflammatory signalling cascade. Excess however can be pro-inflammatory depending on your levels of anti-oxidants.
3. Deal with past hurts and traumas (a very big factor in driving cancer)
4. Reduce outside sources of oestrogen (xeno-estrogens) from your cosmetics, personal care and cleaning products

People with this BRCA gene have been shown to not detoxify well. It is in fact the *gene for DNA repair* and thus if you have the double homozygous variant (one each from both parents), you do not metabolise oestrogens well[ii]. Normally the microbiome helps us to do this if they are healthy, so

---

[i] The most high profile to date was Angelina Jolie but hundreds of other women followed.
[ii] oestrogen requires detoxification to remove them from the body

we need to support the microbiome to do the job. Feed the right food to encourage the ones we want. Prebiotics are actually more important than probiotics i.e. fermented foods and fibre foods.

A recent study by the Mayo clinic implicated the microbiome in breast cancer. However, we now know it's not as simple as that. Remember our genes are interacting (cross-talking) with the genes in our mitos and cells as well as with our environment generally. What is very clear, however, is that removing a breast or other body part is not the answer. You may stave off breast cancer but if toxicity problems remain it will appear somewhere else. And as we will see later in the chapter with German New Medicine (GNM) there are some patterns to where the weak points are and a reasoning.

For now, let's look at some modern innovations which are at least moving us in a direction away from the standard slash and burn therapies.

Modern Innovations in Cancer Therapy

Immunotherapy

Recent innovations have looked at changing the response of the immune system to rogue cells. After all, it is the immune systems job to identify, mark and destroy cancer cells. Many have described cancer as 'an unhealed wound' when looked at from the immunological perspective.[74] It is akin to a loss of central control and, as Thomas Seyfried says that eventually:

"nuclear genomic instability in the tumour cells prevent a return to normal cellular homeostasis. What develops then is an escalating situation of biological chaos, where the intrinsic properties of the immune system (macrophages and local stroma) to *heal wounds* would enhance proliferation in tissue stem cells and their progenitors. Genomic instability and transformation accompany the biological chaos. Collectively, these powerful intrinsic properties drive each other to greater levels of biological disorder and unpredictability all of which arise initially from chronic injury to cellular respiration"[130]

Stem Cell Therapy

A **stem cell** is a cell which has not differentiated yet, it has the potential to become anything. Tumours are known to contain large numbers of these **cancer stem cells (CSCs)** but they are different to normal SCs in that they possess the potential for unlimited growth i.e. are **tumourigenic** cells and are biologically distinct from other subpopulations, being at the top of the hierarchically organised 'tree' of cell types.

As such they are normally considered the reason why conventional treatments may fail or the cancer may 'come back' as they are difficult to eradicate using normal systemic therapies such as irradiation and chemotherapy. They seem immune to the toxicity of such therapies, being more primal. A new approach seeks to target these cells directly; it is called cancer stem cell therapy and is having some interesting results. It is however, still an allopathic (one disease, one treatment) approach.[153]

Fasting and the Fasting Mimicking Diet

Valter Longo and his team in the US have investigated the effect of fasting on cell protection and found that prolonged fasting can "push cells into a highly protected state while making cancer cells highly vulnerable to chemotherapy and other cancer therapies"[154]. However, adherence to the programme of water fasting (i.e. no food) while undergoing the horrors of chemotherapy was understandably not high and so he had to develop a diet that gave all the benefits of fasting without restricting food altogether to encourage people to stick to it. This forms the basis of his 'fasting mimicking diet' (FMD) and represents a 'starvation induced magic shield'. In mice studies this double whammy of FMD and chemo provided a 20-60% cure rate for a variety of cancers even when they had metastasised (spread beyond the original site)[i][155] Not only that but it reduces the side-effects of diarrhoea, pain and hair loss massively —one of the main reasons why chemo is so unpleasant.

These results are revolutionary and as good as immunotherapy. I wonder why this isn't being promoted more by cancer research charities? Could it be that immunotherapy is industry supported and fasting diets are not? Or that oncologists, schooled in the conventional approach, label anything to do with nutrients or food 'unscientific'. That is unfortunate as the results are very well researched[156]. It can help to reduce the chance of recurrence in patients whose cancer is in remission as well as benefit those actively going through chemo. And the benefits are not confined to cancer but

---

[i] But please note the conventional understanding of cancer as a disease that 'spreads (metastasises)' like a virus is a misunderstanding. More likely, cells arise in other parts due to similar issues of toxicity and immunological compromise there.

improvements in blood sugar, cognitive capacity and cellular regeneration generally. But it is not yet 'proven' as far as statutory bodies are concerned so you won't be offered it as standard. You may be able to do a version yourself[i] or as part of a clinical trial however.

Vitamin D Optimisation

Vitamin D is a powerful anti-cancer agent and in fact not a vitamin at all but a powerful pro-hormone formed from cholesterol by the action of sunlight (UVB) on skin. The research is conclusive: low vitamin D levels play a role in the development of all major cancers including breast, prostate, colorectal and even lymphomas. According to recent research the anti-cancer effects are:

1. inhibition of tumour cell proliferation and arrest of the cell cycle
2. induction of apoptosis (programmed cell death) in tumour cells
3. inhibition of invasiveness and angiogenesis (the growth of the tumour's network of blood vessels

Exposure to sunlight is the most efficient way of being Vitamin D optimised. At UK latitudes during March-May and September – October before 11 am and after 3pm, exposing the face, hands and arms for 20- 90 minutes depending on skin type (more for darker skins), equates to about 1000IU/day vitamin D. Required exposure times are substantially less in June to August in the Northern hemisphere (swap this around for Southern hemisphere[ii]). So regular casual exposure of the skin to light[iii] during the cooler hours of the day when the sun's strength his lower should be part of a cancer prevention strategy.

We can absorb vitamin D from foods but it is far less efficient so adding Vitamin D3 (always with K2) as a supplemental intake is vital if you can't access the sun for some reason. However, according to Stepanie Seneff, supplemental or food sources are not quite the same as skin-produced Vitamin D which is sulphated (along with the cholesterol) and it is **cholesterol sulphate (ChS)** which may be the most important molecule –

---

[i] Longo provides extensive notes to oncologists and patients so that they are fully informed.
[ii] Australia in fact has one of the highest incidences of skin cancer – is this because of higher sun exposure, burning (no build up of exposure) and low anti-oxidants?
[iii] It is the ultra-violet (UVB) part of sunlight that produces Vitamin D; it needs to be of a certain frequency. In the winter months the sun is too low in the sky to produce the right frequency. Also clothes, sun lotion and glass all block UVB so we need skin exposure *without* sun block (usually full of toxic chemicals like titanium dioxide and zinc anyhow).

Vit D sulphate is merely the *signalling molecule* that ChS is present in the body[157]. Thus just taking extra vitamin D without the ChS in the skin confuses the body. So letting people out into the sun as a preventative and a palliative strategy is vital. A prescription for sunlight? It may one day happen...

German New Medicine

It would be remiss of me to miss out a very important new understanding of cancer as a result of a **conflict shock** to the body. The originator, lead oncologist Dr. Ryke Hamer, calls this body response to conflict Dirk Hamer Syndrome (DHS – named after his son who died suddenly in a shooting and stimulated his own testicular cancer). Dr Hamer has developed a theory that cancer is the body's response of enacting a **Significant Biological Special Programme (SBS)** designed to *heal* that conflict, not a disease. This approach is called German New Medicine®[i].

This work was developed from both his own personal experience but developed as he was an oncologist and could therefore study CT scans of brains of people with cancer and map what parts of the brain were stimulated and correlating with the type of conflict shock they'd had and the type of cancer they developed. He identified many different types of conflict from separation, abandonment, isolation, feeling attacked, etc. and saw that there were consistent reactions in the same parts of the brain and then bodies of those people. Thus he developed a theory that is now known as the 5 Biological Laws.

In the first law he determined that the reactions follow a particular trajectory over 3 different levels of expression:

1. Psyche – your subjective experience i.e. the meaning of what happens determined by cultural, familial conditioning – individual for each person.
2. Brain – the area of the brain corresponding to the type of conflict e.g. specific areas of the cortex, brainstem, limbic system, etc.
3. Organ – the function of a particular organ associated with that brain region e.g. breast, lung, prostate, etc.

In the second law he mapped out the two phases of the SBS – the first is the conflict active phase identified by **sympathetic dominance** (fight and flight) and the second by **parasympathetic dominance** or **vagotonia** as he calls it. There will always be a healing crisis which the body induces to

---

[i] See http://www.newmedicine.ca/ for more information and resources.

resolve this second phase which is where symptoms are perceived; they may be the tumour in cancer or indeed a cold[i], migraine, body pain, heart attack, etc in other illnesses. Most people get stuck here as modern medicine treats the symptom only and will suppress the body's attempt at resolution.

The third law links the ontogenesis (also sometimes called morphogenesis) which is 'the origination and development of an organism, usually from the time of fertilization of the egg to the organism's mature form[158]' to the type of cancer you may form. This understanding of the development of the embryo and how it maps to the adult human brain has much in common with the triune brain model which I expounded earlier in Chapter Four but adds a whole new dimension to the idea of birth and childhood trauma.

The fourth law states that: there is a correspondence between the embryonic layer-related organ groups – and groups of microbes that are mobilised to resolve the problem in the healing phase.

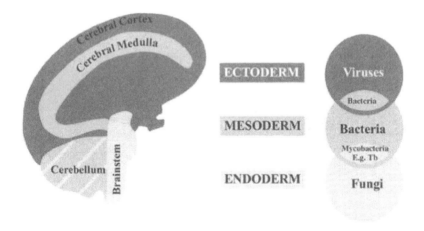

Figure 50: Mapping the Brain to Microbe Correlation ©GNM

It is now recognised that the embryo that you once were *stores evolutionary memory* in its tissues that go way beyond your experience as a person. Indeed, if this seems far-fetched let m e just remind you, biology has never been fully able to explain how the foetus is programmed to develop in the way it does, though some believe this is a quantum process[ii].

---

[i] In some bizarre cases cancer has been cured by the body mounting a response to a cold or flu virus. I kid you not. This approach might explain such anomalies.

The fifth law summarises all the previous ones by stating that basically disease (even cancer) is *explainable* and not random – that all diseases have a special biological meaning. There is much more to say about this theory that I can't go into here but I've tried to summarise in the diagram below. But suffice to say it offers a new model of cancer – not as a disease but as a *programmed response of the body to self-heal.*

I urge you to investigate this new understanding at the very least to break the stranglehold of fear which encircles this subject. When we adopt this understanding we are encouraged to treat our cancer not with toxic drugs but with things that support the body's natural healing mechanisms. I find that idea hugely inspiring and hope it will develop more powerful treatments in future as it develops though it is controversial and disputed[i].

Table 4: New German Medicine Summary

Embryo Part	Brain part	Conflicts	Body part	Microbe
Endoderm	Brainstem (digestion and breath).	Death fright (breathing, nourishment conflict	Lungs, gut, uterus	Fungi
Old Mesoderm	Cerebellum (protection/ support)	Nurture/ connection	Breast glands	Bacteria
Young mesoderm	Cerebral medulla	Self devaluation	muscles, bones and ligaments	Bacteria
Ectoderm	Cerebral cortex	social /sexual/separation	Breast ducts.	Viruses

Summary

Real progress in cancer management and prevention will emerge once the cancer field abandons the somatic mutation theory and comes to recognise

---

ii Prof. Rupert Sheldrake has looked at this extensively in his 'A New Science of Life'.
i While researching this I became aware that two different authors are currently writing under the supposed auspices of Dr Hamer and, as he died in 2017, the dispute continues.

the role of the mitochondria in the origin, management, and prevention of the disease. Your cells pick up the message of threat from your environment and this is translated into the cell danger response and the shift to oxidative glycolysis. We need to look at the biopsychosocial environment of the person with cancer and change those parameters that can be changed – good food, more sunlight, social connection and laughter. Cancer, like other diseases is best not seen in isolation from the person who has it. We need to know what their life history has been and how they perceive their world as well as what symptoms they have.

Chapter 9: Mind and Body in Healthy Ageing

If, as we now believe, the brain is no longer considered the heart of consciousness, if in fact it exists throughout all matter, particularly in an organised system such as the cell and the microstructures within the cell, then we need to stop looking in the brain or organ for the origin of all disease and consider instead the intricate body systems and beyond to our interaction with our environment. One final aspect of the complexity of the human interaction with the wider environment is an area I've left til last as it is perhaps the most esoteric (although has very good data to support it). This area includes the fields of chronobiology and quantum coherence.

Chronobiology: Light, Time and the Rhythms of Life

We have evolved as a species in response to the rhythms of the earth. The most potent of those is the cycle of light and dark. Throughout our evolution (until the last 100 years or so with the advent of electric light) we would have risen with the sun and gone to bed not long after sunset with only the moon and stars, a candle or the light of a fire to see by. Our brains and bodies have evolved methods to interact with that light to control our metabolic processes. Indeed our internal time-clock which naturally runs on a 25 hour cycle has to be synchronised each morning with daylight to bring it back to a 24 hour one. So early morning daylight helps our body know what time of day it is and to begin daytime processes.

We have long known that our brains are sensitive to light via the optic nerve to the eyes. But recently a very specific part called the **suprachiasmatic nucleus** (**SCN**[i] - the master clock) has been discovered which connects with the **pineal gland** to release melatonin which regulates

---

[i] just above where the optic nerves cross = chiasm hence the name suprachiasmatic nucleus

sleep/wake cycles. A burst of sunlight in the morning sets the cycle going into its normal rhythm of going up at night and down just before daylight (circadian rhythm).

The SCN registers the time of day by the quality of light that the retina receives – more blue in the morning and redder towards sunset and at night (from the light of a fire). This pattern has continued for thousands of years and it deeply rooted in our physiology. However, since the industrial revolution, we have circumvented this normal pattern with electric light allowing us to stay up far beyond sunset and often having to force ourselves up before sunrise. Recent developments of low energy LED bulbs have made this situation far worse as this light is very bright white (no infra red as in incandescent bulbs) thus containing a tiny portion of the full spectrum of daylight which fools our body into thinking it's the middle of the day in the evening! This has consequences: most of us are stressed and sleep deprived from being somewhat insomniac.

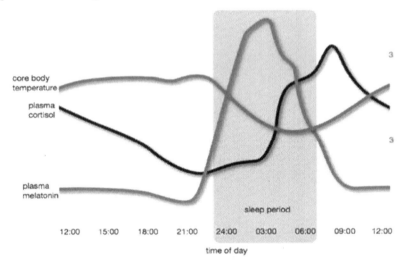

Figure 51: Circadian and Cortisol Cycle Synchronicity

Melatonin normally increases over the night during slow-wave sleep, but it is not only a sleep hormone. It actually suppresses insulin during the night to keep blood glucose available during the 8-10 hour fast for all the night-time processes of clearance of toxins, etc. Not only that but it primes our immune system too via the T-Regs. So lack of sleep not only affects our sleep and mood but our immune functioning too. It is not only the SCN which picks up light but the **paraventricular nucleus (PVN)** of the **hypothalamus** (the stress response system), connects with the hippocampus and stimulates cortisol release to raise blood sugar and keep us active. So, according to Dr Datis Kharrazian, "in order to be healthy the pineal (melatonin) and hippocampal/hypothalamic (cortisol) pathways must synchronise". The rise in cortisol is what wakes us up!

Few people realise that the skin is a light sensitive organ too. We know that it's essential for Vitamin D production but did you know that ultra-violet light (UVA) in contact with the skin releases **ACTH (adrenocorticotropic hormone)** - the cortisol-stimulating hormone that wakes us up and gets us moving[159]? This is a very recent finding. We used to think only the pituitary released that. Our skin is therefore tied to the sun cycle too. It, along with the light entering our eyes, help control the release of cortisol to regulate our energy so that we have a peak in the morning and then gradually lowering over the day to promote sleepiness.

The eyes are particularly adapted to light – the retina is a form of inverted skin which transfers light down the optic nerve to the pineal to release melatonin as we've already discussed. But how it does this is a very interesting chemical reaction where it creates an intermediated heparin sulphate during the day when exposed to natural daylight. This sulphate is then passed to melatonin when the light dims in the evening to allow the melatonin to be made soluble in the watery cerebro-spinal fluid. So, according to Stephanie Seneff, you can get a deficiency in melatonin because of a lack of available sulphate from sun exposure to the eyes. Even though you have enough melatonin, if it can't be made soluble it's unable to do its job.

Many modern people in Western nations hardly expose themselves to natural sunlight (UVA doesn't transmit through a window) and their circadian rhythm gets very distorted with sleepiness in the morning and a burst of energy in the evening when they should be going to bed (common particularly in teenagers and people with fatigue syndromes).

Eating late at night has a direct effect on this as it promotes digestion which steals energy from what the body should be doing at night which is basically repair and recycling of damaged cells and cellular parts (autophagy). This requires a fasting state and thus eating for longer over the day (feeding window) has the effect of dysregulating our hormones (particularly cortisol). I talked about this much more in my last book, the World Within, but extending your **fasting window**[i] from 10 – 14 hours has huge benefits for cellular efficiency. Regular mealtimes are also important to keep this cycles entrained. The brain is always trying to predict patterns and if you disrupt this by eating earlier one day from another, (or skipping breakfast altogether some days) this creates an issue. Your mitochondria and gut bacteria are also attuned to time of day, season and even moon phases so eating seasonally (with more carbs like berries and root veg in the autumn and winter), and foods that your grandparents would recognize (so you are genetically adapted to) is also important.

Light Therapy

There is another reaction that occurs when sunlight tans the skin; it is actually causing a photochemical reaction with tyrosine in the skin forming dark-pigmented **melanin**. Along with chemical conversion of vitamin D, we can thus surmise that light can be absorbed by the skin to enact chemical reactions. We also know it can turn genes on and off now using light in a process called **optogenetics** so by using certain frequencies of red light for instance you can improve your sleep and cellular functioning.

Hot and Cold Therapy

Endorphins are released when we experience heat and cold (like sauna and cold showers) and helps to build resilience. It is the basis of natural therapy called contrast bathing/hydrotherapy but is now very trendy as cryotherapy – where you bathe in ice cold water for a few minutes before heating up the body again. The benefits also stem from cellular changes due to heat shock proteins which we discussed in Chapter 3. It is a hormetic stressor (remember hormesis) which in small amounts improves the health of our mitochondria.

Heart Coherence and Quantum Biology

According to Gregg Braden the heart has its own nervous system consisting of **sensory neurites**. Work by the HeartMath Institute has investigated this system that allows the heart to pick up information just like the brain (in

---

[i] Although this doesn't suit everyone, it's still a good general rule to not snack late at night. People with the ApoE4 gene variant should fast for longer.

fact ahead of the brain). It's linked to the heart coherence we looked at in Chapter 3. So could the heart also be a 'mind' too? That's a very interesting question and I refer you to the detailed data from HeartMath Institute which shows that people can synchronise with the shifting magnetic rhythms of the earth, albeit unconsciously[160]. Those that don't are likely disconnected physiologically from the earth that gave them life and are doing a great deal of damage to themselves and others. The head of HeartMath Rollin McCraty warns us against becoming disconnected from our connection with earth energy and our hearts.

The heart and the brain are in direct communication but it's 90% from *heart to brain* rather than the other way round. When our heart is in coherence we gain more mental clarity, flow and a sense of wonder and connectedness. And these abilities are our birthright but we may never have been shown how to develop these skills by our parents or elders as the understanding has been lost by our culture.

Mindbody Concepts and a New Paradigm of Healing

There is a new understanding which we are (re-) discovering about the nature of the mindbody as an energetic being, independent of the material world which it inhabits. This information was known about by ancient peoples but was largely lost over the centuries as vested interests have edited the information available to us. But modern experiments at the cutting edge of physics could be about to revive some of this knowledge. Indeed this is where science and the spiritual traditions can be said to interact and inform eachother. Some of this information has direct effects on how our body interacts with time and space (the basis of ageing). To paraphrase Harvard scientist and researcher Marilyn Shlitz[i]:

"It is at the meeting place of science and spiritual wisdom that we discover a new paradigm, which sheds light on aging" gracefully or even, 'gratefully'! To engage in our own positive transformation requires cultivating a positive healing and 'growth-oriented mindset'"[161]

It is not just about 'fixing the problem' whether from a conventional or alternative view. They are both allopathic concepts. In the new model we consider that all things are connected and interdependent. Medicine is still

---

[i] She co-produced the film 'Death Makes Life Possible' with Deepak Chopra. See her website marilynschlitz.com

taught in the 20th century mindset of Newtonian physics and mechanical interactions and it's time to update the programme to one that is more holistic, and quantum. In my first book I looked at some new concepts in health science that are overturning the old view:

Table 5: New Concepts in Health Science

1. Brain plasticity (neuroplasticity/growth) is now known to occur throughout life; we adapt our neuronal function depending on environment. Health is a continuum and the body is a complex system that operates as a whole not parts; as a system not organ-based model.
2. 'Disease is a manifestation of a dysfunctional system'[162]of which genetic predisposition is a part not the whole – and it is a dynamic interplay which shifts genes on and off (epigenetics not a fixed programme)Mind seems to be a non-local (not limited to space-time) concept; a hologram of universal consciousness, independent of the brain. This is now established science in the world of physics[163] but not yet in medicine.
3. Our adverse childhood experiences (ACE) have huge physiological effects throughout our life due to a change in our brain's and therefore our cell's stress response[164].
4. Our ancestors' experiences also shape who we are via the epigenetic transmission of DNA variation – largely through the microbiome and mitochondria'

The study of epigenetics has shown us that "we have the ability to change the way our DNA is expressed – through epigenetic changes, largely mediated via our microbiome and mitochondria (both microbial in origin) but originating in consciousness. Mind permeates our whole being including our cells. They could truly be said to be *intelligent*.

Complexity Theory Within Living Systems

Complexity theory says that within any system that has complexity there will also be randomness, chaos or unpredictability. However, it develops adaptation as an *emergent property* to the problems presented to it over time. These changes tend towards the furthering if its own evolution i.e. biofeedback changes within the system allow growth, learning and creativity. Thus natural systems are *dynamic informational exchange not random machines.*

Consciousness is the foundation of this chaos system which makes it simultaneously:

1. Sentient (it can sense the surroundings via sensory feedback)
2. Unitary/ complementary (mind and matter are one and equivalent)

178

3. Recursive (it feeds back to engender higher order)

So the purpose of nature, you could say, is evolution, higher order, self-awareness, and enlightenment. Biologically speaking, every cell has a purpose different from other cells but all belong to a higher order of being, a whole. It is the development of the whole through the parts that are evolving. Perhaps this is purpose enough.

Don't forget the mind and body are one. So the thoughts you think and the life you live are intimately connected with your body's cellular responses (as I've already demonstrated in Chapter 6 with values). It's the thesis of this entire book really but it still a new paradigm. An energetic (quantum physics-based concept of health) has been largely ignored by medical science. We know that concepts of quantum biology such as "entanglement, called 'spooky action at a distance' by Albert Einstein, may also exist at the macro-level of human beings (and not just at the micro-level of subatomic particles)"[165]. They certainly exist within our cells and energy healing and remote viewing show us that health isn't all about the physical interventions and matter as the basis of life. As Marilyn Schlitz, says:

"It is time to challenge our cultural assumptions about aging. By shifting our worldview from fear to inspiration, we can see this demographic shift—and our place in it—as an opportunity for immense personal and collective growth and transformation. As each of us confronts aging—our own or that of others—we find creative ways of living and being in the world. We sense that there is more to our existence—more layers or dimensions than we comprehend in our daily lives. For some, this awakens an embrace of meaning and purpose fostering our kinship—or interconnectedness—with a greater whole. Many of us speak up for a new model of aging conceived as a great awakening".

Quantum Concepts in a Cellular World

Up to now most molecular and biological science has been focused on the material realm i.e. 'things'. But, as I've alluded to already there is a new understanding of matter that takes its cue from quantum physics that matter is not primary but a function of energy or information. Specifically, the idea that not only light can exist as a wave or particle[i] but biological molecules too e.g. DNA, RNA and most proteins is just beginning to be acknowledged in cutting-edge research. That mainstream science hasn't

---

[i] Wave/particle duality of light as it is termed was discovered in the 1920s but was thought to be exclusive to non-biological phenomena

accepted this yet is only due to the silo nature of medicine and physics; they are worlds apart.

One aspect recently discussed by eminent researcher Sungchul Ji is the idea of the importance of quantum waves in cell function:

"Cell language is defined as the language living cells use to communicate with one another or within themselves employing molecules as words and texts. One of the predictions made by the cell language theory (CLT) is that there are two forms of genetic information – the Watson-Crick genes transmitting information in time (identified with DNA), and the Prigoginian[i] genes transmitting information in space (identified with RNA expression profiles). The former is analogous to sheet music or written language and the latter is akin to audio music or spoken language, both being coupled by **conformons** acting as the analog of the pianist. [166]

So let's just explain that really important understanding for a minute. What he is saying is that the DNA blueprint is like sheet music which can be interpreted in many different ways by a different pianist to produce the music as language. Think for a moment the difference between a virtuoso and an inexperienced pianist. They both read the same 'language' but the results are spectacularly different. It is in the reading (to RNA) that the cell function will alter not the blueprint per se. And this is an informational (wave) function of biological molecules which he terms 'conformons' to describe the "conformational wave packet in biopolymers carrying both the free energy and genetic information."[167]

But how do these conformons receive the information to begin their transformation? He maintains it is activation of these complex molecules *with energy* that primes them to engage in work much like a battery charge enables a battery to drive a machine. For example, with DNA it has long been known that it has to be **supercoiled** in order to be expressed into RNA. An enzyme called DNA gyrase splits the DNA strand, adds a twist into the chain by rotating it along its length so adding energy into the system (much like winding the spring of a clock or watch). It is this energy that allows the gene (a specific section of the DNA) to be expressed by attracting the relevant enzymes that open up the DNA coil and transcribe

---

[i] Ilya Prigogine, a physical chemist who received the Nobel Prize in 1977 for contributions to non-equilibrium thermodynamics as applied to complex systems including living organisms. His work is fundamental to the new disciplines of complexity and chaos theories.

the bases into RNA. This is something that is very hard to explain in a materialist way. See the diagram overleaf for more explanation.

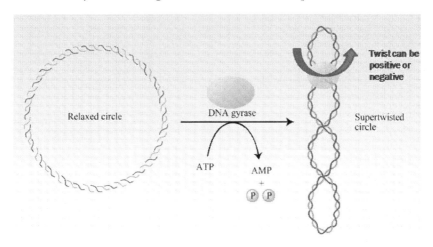

Figure 52: DNA as a Conformon

How does the enzyme 'know' which bit to approach? Now we have an answer that it is the *stored energy* in that part of the sequence that concentrates the enzymes at that point something called **'stress-induced duplex destabilisation' (SIDD)**.[168] Don't worry that these terms may be new to you – they are to most people outside of the esoteric fields of computational biology! The important thing to note is that DNA is not just a physical structure but an energetic/informational one.

We also know that there are 3 types of waveforms that operate in cells:

1. Light
2. Sound
3. Concentration

The last one is of particular interest for us as it is where certain concentration gradients are set up which allow for cellular functioning e.g. concentration of calcium ions from the nucleus to the membrane which changes its function. Waves, unlike particles can transcend physical barriers (like radiowaves do), they can interfere with each other (like ripples on a pond), and they can theoretically flow outwards infinitely allowing very distant points to communicate ('action at a distance'). This allows for such conundrums as remote healing: if it is a wave form that controls certain cellular functioning, then it is not beyond the realms of possibility that the social environment of human to human interaction would change the DNA expression too. This 'field of research that examines why and how different social factors and processes (e.g., social stress, internal conflict, isolation, attachment, etc.) affect the activity of the genome is termed **sociogenomics** and it is a relatively new but promising field[169].

DNA as an Informational Molecule

We have already touched on this in previous chapters but here I would like to describe three experiments on DNA which challenge our view of the material world as isolated and random.

The first was by a Russian scientist Vladmir Poponin who isolated human DNA in a vacuum tube and found that when removing the DNA the photons (the smallest 'packet' of light) present in the tube were ordered – they retained a memory of the DNA even though it wasn't physically present. The summary of this by the scientist was that DNA is communicating with the quantum world via an invisible quantum field.or 'matrix' as some have termed it. This is termed the 'phantom DNA' experiment.

The second experiment conducted by the US Army under researcher Dr Cleve Backster put human DNA in a device that could measure its responsiveness and put the donor into another separate room. Then they subjected the donor to emotional stimulation while measuring the DNA. The separated DNA matched the emotional peaks and troughs of the donor *instantaneously* as measured by an atomic clock – and this experiment has been replicated hundreds of miles apart. This suggests that emotions are communicating with our DNA *non-locally* i.e. it is everywhere not located in space time. The only way this can be explained is if they are "still connected in some way" and the quantum field or matrix is thereby invoked again as the most likely explanation.

The third experiment was conducted by the Institute of HeartMath. Human DNA was isolated to observe changes in the presence of heart-based emotion and showed when there were coherent emotions of love, rage, etc. In the presence of positive appreciation, love and forgiveness DNA became very relaxed and this promoted a good immune response via opening up the portions of DNA that benefited immunity. With the opposite emotions of hate, anger and fear DNA became compressed and immunity was decreased. Thus emotion has the power to change the shape and function of DNA within our bodies. We might think of this as a new internal technology.

So, as a summary:

1. DNA is not fixed in its material form. It connects with a connective field or matrix of energy that connects any one thing with everything else in the universe.
2. The DNA in our bodies gives us access to the energy that connects our universe, and emotion is the key to tapping in to the field.

As Dr. Jeffrey Thompson, a colleague of Cleve Backster, states so eloquently, from this viewpoint: "there is no place where one's body actually ends and no place where it begins." Perhaps it also explains some of the ancient healing texts which talk about the power of the mind to alter the body. I leave you with the words of Poponin himself:

"We believe this discovery has tremendous significance for the explanation and deeper understandings of the mechanisms underlying subtle energy phenomena including many of the observed alternative healing phenomena."

Remember these are respected physical scientists saying this. This is no longer the preserve of the irrational and esoteric (even though there was a lot of wisdom in those teachings).

Towards a Cellular View of Health

I hope I have shown you the wonder and magnificence of our biology and that, with knowledge and appropriate lifestyle change, we *can talk to our cells* in a way that removes the blocks to healing and increases our longevity. Our body and the diseases we get are not our body trying to harm us but *keep us alive*. Dysfunction is a lack of balance in the whole and we would do well to remember this when treating symptoms like cancer or Alzheimer's disease[i]. Treatments that simply manage the symptoms do nothing to address the underlying cause and keep the patient stuck, depending on expensive drugs and surgeries that can deepen suffering.

That's not to say that technology has no place in our healthcare. Some of the innovations I have described in this book are simply amazing and help to prolong life. However, I do question extending lifespan without

---

[i] As author of The Longevity Diet, Valter Longo says 'it's like trying to improve a Beethoven symphony by adding more cellos'. I liked that analogy. You can't tinker with parts.

healthspan. What is the point of living longer lives when we are full of pain and dysfunction? We need to seek rational but also somewhat 'out of the box' solutions to what is a system of amazing complexity and diversity. No one person can heal the same way as another, as indeed no one disease has the same precedent in everyone. But by tackling the common issues of dysbiosis (gut imbalance), autonomic dysfunction and toxicity we can all get good results.

We are finding our current medical system inadequate for the vast majority of patients because it does not train its doctors in a holistic systems approach but looks at bits or parts (called 'specialties' in medical training). The focus is then on which bits might fail randomly requiring expensive technological solutions (usually drugs or surgery) keeping the vast majority of people suffering chronic illness. This model is bankrupting our economies and wasting the energies of our medical students who become disillusioned doctors with high levels of addiction, burn-out and consequent early retirement. Functional medicine is a new approach that may yet save us but it can't come soon enough as the current focus on disease rather than health is crippling the healthcare system[i].

A true health service looks at the body as a wondrous cellular feedback system and we the patient become active, energised, *empowered* participants in the process of healing. And it uses natural lifestyle means to achieve cellular health: detoxification, good food, exercise, sleep, sunshine and stress release to do it[170]. Roll on the next revolution!

Final Thoughts

When we connect with the wonder and complexity of cellular selves, we educate and empower ourselves to step forward as humans taking responsibility for our inner and outer worlds. For, at a biomolecular level, we are all one as we interchange microbes and molecules with our biosphere. I have hoped to show you (perhaps in too much detail!) how amazing our cells and their interconnectivity are to inspire you to take charge, get educated, and send your cells the message of love that they deserve. Your reward is true health – it may not be easy, but nothing worthwhile ever is.

---

[i] Of the $3trillion US spend on healthcare only 5% is on prevention. Likely the UK is similar.

Epilogue

My first book, The Scar that Won't Heal (revised 2017) was a labour of love when I knew nothing about how to write a book or get it published. I eventually chose the self-publishing option as it enabled me to get it out sooner (getting a non-fiction book on the subject of trauma written when you are neither a world-class scientist nor a journalist with connections, is hard!). But I did it and continue to get good feedback. My second, The World Within in 2017, had me polishing my publishing skills to then revisit the first book and add an index and improve the layout and look. Finally book 3 – this one – is here and I feel I have done more than most to present to you the full complexity of the story of our cellular selves. This is cutting edge information I have gleaned from hundreds of hours of study. I may have dazzled you with science but I hope I have also ignited in you a quest to learn more and take charge of your health and wellbeing.

Last year (2018), I set to recording an audio book version of The Scar that Won't Heal, little knowing how difficult that would be. Hundreds of hours and a few thousand pounds later I am nearing completion of that. It has given me the idea to produce more audio content for people who don't want to or can't access the written material. I am always studying and learning in order to better understand what makes us humans tick. This latest project aims to get this information more widely out there so that people can heal themselves with a little information and support. In order to do this I need to free up some time from my 1-2-1 client work to be able to produce more podcasts and videos with some of this vital information.

With the help of online platform Patreon I am hoping to get sponsorship from you, the interested public. Please visit my Patreon page for details of how you can sign up for regular exclusive content – and even get yourself name-checked in my next book! **www.patreon.com/patriciaworby**

I would be delighted to hear from you and, if you enjoyed the book do get in touch and, better still please **leave me a review on my amazon page**.

Thank you for your support.

Further reading

Books

Here is a short selection of essential books on the subject. I have limited it to those I have personally read and found helpful and specifically deal with longevity and cellular ageing. A much wider reading list is given via references throughout the text.

- Jeffrey Bland. The Disease Delusion
- Bruce Lipton. The Biology of Belief
- Valter Longo, The Longevity Diet
- Ben Lynch, Dirty Genes
- Candace Pert,. The Molecules of Emotion
- Terry L. Wahls Minding My Mitochondria

Websites

- www.alchemytherapies.co.uk
- www.drperlmutter.com
- www.ifm.org
- https://jeffreybland.com/
- www.geneticlifehacks.com

Glossary of terms

Here I include the essential concepts relevant to our discussion that occur more than once in this text. There are many important terms I have defined within these pages but if they occur only once I have not referenced them here although I have italicised them for emphasis.

Adenosine triphosphate (ATP) - molecule of energy production and a signalling molecule produced throughout the body in the cell mitochondria.

Allostasis – the point of chemical equilibrium in the body in which we function most well - formerly called homeostasis.

Allostatic load - the sum total of all the physical, chemical and psychological stresses on the body.

Antioxidant - compounds (e.g. glutathione, Vitamin C)that inhibit oxidation and quench reactive oxygen species.

Auto-immune disease (AID) - a category of diseases consisting of immune over stimulation where the body mistakenly attacks its own tissues believing them to be foreign. Many examples exist e.g. Rheumatoid arthritis and Hashimoto's thyroiditis.

Autonomic nervous system (ANS) – part of our nervous system (alongside the CNS below) that works behind the scenes to regulate our body without our conscious involvement such as breathing, the heartbeat, and digestion. It has two branches the sympathetic (fight and flight) and para-sympathetic (rest and digest). It is mainly efferent i.e. body to brain.

Autophagy – the natural intracellular degradation mechanism by which cells (and organelles like mitochondria) renew themselves in order to recycle their materials and keep functioning efficiently

Blood Brain Barrier (BBB) - a highly selective semi-permeable membrane barrier that separates the circulating blood from the brain extracellular fluid in the brain. Keeps the brain free of toxins.

Brain-gut-microbiota axis (BGM) – the very important neuro-endocrine links between these three organs which co-ordinate responses to the environment. Highly implicated in health and disease.

Cachexia – the loss of weight common with cancer due to hyper-fermentation of glucose leading to uncontrolled cell proliferation and tumourigenesis

Central Nervous System (CNS) – one of the two branches of nervous system with the autonomic nervous system. This consists of primarily the voluntary functions and is mainly afferent i.e. brain to body through the spinal cord.

Chelator - a molecule that binds minerals – used by the body to detoxify and remove toxins from the body. Examples include chlorella (an algae) and DSM (an organic chemical).

Chromosome - the tightly wound DNA pairs in the nucleus of the cell. 1 from each parent creates biological variation.

Chromophore - a chemical high in double bonds that helps harvest light and provides food with its colouring.

Cytochrome P450 (CYP) enzyme - a very important detoxification enzyme in the liver, the strength of which varies depending on your genetic make-up.

Cytokines – small signalling molecules such as interferon, interleukin, and growth factors, secreted by certain cells of the immune system

Cytoplasm (cytosol) the cell fluid surrounding the nucleus. Contains dissolved solutes and proteins.

Diabetes – a disease of blood sugar dyregulation due to overwhelm of the cell to the hormone insulin. See also insulin resistance.

Deoxyribonucleic Acid (DNA) – the genetic code of life consisting of 4 bases (the letters) Adenine (A), Guanine (G), Cytosine (C) and Thymine (T)

Dysbiosis – a general term to describe the imbalance of gut flora which contributes to disease. Hippocrates, the father of medicine, said 'all disease begins in the gut' and this is now corroborated.

Electron Transport Chain (ETC) - a chain of protein complexes in the inner membrane of a mitochondrion that allow energy production by transfer of electrons, protons and photons.

Enteric nervous system (ENS) - the nerve complexes that line the gut – also called the 'gut-brain'. Mostly consisting of efferent (towards the brain) fibres.

Epigenetics - the study of the factors above the simple reading of genetic blueprint which dictates what genes are read and in what order. Factors include diet, tissue pH, stress hormones and so on.

Functional medicine - a systems-based model of medicine that looks at rebalancing the inter-relationships between hormonal, neuronal, nutritional systems of the body. It seeks to identify and address the root causes of disease rather than simply treat symptoms. Although, not the conventional view yet, it is rapidly gaining ground and will, no doubt, be the future of medicine .

Free radicals or **Reactive Oxygen Species (ROS)** - an uncharged molecule (typically highly reactive and short-lived) with an unpaired electron; ROS are free radicals of oxygen like specifically involving oxygen like peroxide, superoxide, etc.

Genome complexity conundrum – the surprising finding that human genome contained only 26,000 genes – roughly the same as an earthworm! Our complexity has been subsequently found to be due to contribution of the microbiome.

Genotype – the particular configuration of genes that an individual has i.e. its genetic makeup.

Glial cells - specialised caretaker cells that insulate and help neurones in the brain keep healthy.

Histones – the protein wrapping around DNA that keeps it stable and free from damage. Has to be unravelled whenever the DNA needs to be read.

Homeostasis – tendency towards a relatively stable equilibrium between interdependent elements, especially as maintained by physiological processes within the body.

Horizontal gene transfer (HGT) is the movement of genetic material between unicellular and/or multicellular organisms compared to the more widely understood 'vertical transmission' (the transmission of DNA from parent to offspring). Probably so named because genetic family trees are normally mapped vertically for the parents and horizontally for the offspring.

Human Genome Project, launched in 1990, is a project that would fully map and sequence the human genome. It completed in 2003.

Inflammation – the natural process by which the body defends itself against attack or damage via the release of pro-inflammatory cytokines. Characterised by redness, swelling and fever in acute form, but can become chronic if not regulated which results in disease.

Insulin resistance – the result of too much insulin on the cell membrane is to reduce the number of receptors so that the cell becomes resistant to insulin.

Intestinal permeability (leaky gut) – finally accepted by mainstream medicine as contributing to disease, this syndrome of opening up of the gut barrier allows proteins to enter into the bloodstream causing the immune system to react to food as if it were a pathogen and mount an immune response.

Ligand – the chemical messenger that attaches to the outside receptor of a cell to stimulate a chemical change inside the cell

Matrisome, the term given to all the components of the ECM consisting of extracellular fluid, mast cells and tunnel-like structures called fibroblasts.

Metabolomics – the study of the set of metabolites (cellular protein, lipid and other macromolecule content) present within an organism, cell, or tissue. A chemical 'signature', in other words, brought about by advances in detection methods

Microbiome – the collective name for the microbes that live in and on your body – specifically it refers to the DNA component (microbial genome) but has now come to mean the organisms themselves.

Microtubules - microscopic tubular structure present in the cytoplasm of cells which acts as scaffolding and can organise to pull apart the cell during cell division

Mitochondria – organelles (small components) of the cell which produce energy by means of respiration (burning of glucose using oxygen to produce ATP.

Mitochondriopathy – a failure of the mitochondria to produce enough energy due to down-regulation of the system by toxicity and stress. At the heart of most chronic disease including cancer.

Neuropeptides – small protein molecules that, like neurotransmitters, communicate information throughout the body.

Neuroplasticity - the term given to the modification of neuronal pathways in the brain (the chain of nerve cells) as a result of changes in the environment. Now known to occur throughout life.

Non-communicable disease (NCD) — new designation for chronic types of disease now seen more prevalently than the communicable (infectious) types of disease that used to afflict mankind. We tend not to die from them but they are the leading cause of death worldwide, which modern medicine struggles to solve.

Oxidative phosphorylation (or **oxphos**) — a series of chemical reactions in the mitochondria that use oxygen to produce energy from glucose via the electron transport chain. The most efficient way of producing energy for the body.

Phenotype -the set of observable characteristics of an individual resulting from the interaction of its genotype with the environment.

Photosynthesis — the process by which plants make energy from sunlight using carbon dioxide and releasing oxygen. Uses chlorophyll in the leaves.

Prebiotic - a carbohydrate that probiotic microbes preferentially eat.

Psychobiotics —a group of probiotic bacteria, which, when ingested, confer mental health benefits through interactions with commensal gut bacteria.

Psychoneuroimmunology - the study of the interaction between psychological processes and the nervous and immune systems of the human body.

Receptors — proteins embedded in the membranes of cells (and sometimes in the cytosol) which bind to certain molecules like the lock and key to trigger a molecular action.

Single nucleotide polymorphism (SNiP) — unlike mutations which involve whole genes, this is a small change in the DNA alphabet of bases that has one base alteration (letter). Very common and can now be mapped to give an indication of your susceptibility to certain conditions.

Stress response — a specific physiological hormonal and neurological response to perturbations of the internal and external environment to bring it back into homeostasis.

Th1 or Th2 dominant immunity — reflects the type of T-helper cells that predominate in your immune response (roughly correlating to whether the innate or adaptive type immune systems). Th1 type cytokines produce the pro-inflammatory responses responsible for killing intracellular microbes and cancer and Th2 cells are anti-inflammatory and aim to destroy pathogens that occur outside our cells (bacteria and parasites). Imbalance in either of these branches tends to result in auto-immune disease or cancer respectively.

Vagus Nerve —very important parasympathetic nerve (originating 10th Cranial nerve of brainstem) which regulates organs above and below the diaphragm; ventral vagal (VV) and dorsal vagal (DV) respectively. Also called 'the wanderer'

ABOUT THE AUTHOR

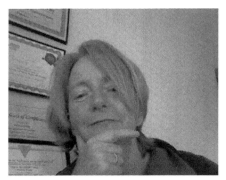

Patricia Worby, PhD, MSc. is a former scientist, now researcher and specialist practitioner in chronic fatigue and pain. She worked for the NHS for 15 years and currently the University of Southampton for 10 years in clinical research and latterly as a Research Manager. After graduation she was going to 'change the world through science' but life intervened in a quite surprising way. After a series of health challenges in her 30's, including depression and chronic fatigue, she was encouraged to find her own answers and is now a passionate advocate of natural medicine. Today, she is a trauma therapist who specialises in chronic illness especially ME/CFS and Fibromyalgia using a holistic approach to nutrition, massage and emotional healing. Her PhD is in the correlations between unresolved implicit memory and chronic pain.

She can be found at www.patriciaworby.co.uk (general writing, speaking and educational site) and www.alchemytherapies.co.uk (clinic site)

References

1 Bland, Jeffrey. The Disease Delusion; conquering the causes of chronic illness for a healthier, longer and happier life. Harper Collins 2014 P178

2 Hamilton, G. (2014). The Micromanagers. New Scientist, 223(2987), 42-45.

3Worby, Patricia (2018rev). The World Within; how your microbiome makes you who you are. Kdp/ Createspace

4 Gibney E. (2019). How 'magic angle' graphene is stirring up science. Nature. 565 16-18

5Sinatra ST, et al (2017). Electric Nutrition: The Surprising Health and Healing Benefits of Biological Grounding (Earthing). Altern. Ther. Health Med. Sep;23(5):8-16.

6Naba, Alexandra et al. (2011)Thematrisome: in silico definition and in vivo characterization by proteomics of normal and tumour extracellular matrices. Mol. Cell Proteomics Dec 9, mcp.M111.014647; https://doi.org/10.1074/mcp.

7 Duncan, Georgina. (2108). Fascia: its role in Health and Cancer. Exmouth Wellness Centre Blog. August 17

8Philpott, HT (2017). Attenuation of early phase inflammation by cannabidiol prevents pain and nerve damage in rat osteoarthritis. Pain. Dec;158(12):2442-2451. doi: 10.1097/j.pain.0000000000001052.

9Jurkus R (2016) Cannabidiol Regulation of Learned Fear: Implications for Treating Anxiety-Related Disorders. Front Pharmacol. Nov 24;7:454. eCollection

10Scallan, J. et al.. (2016). Lymphatic pumping: mechanics, mechanisms and malfunction. J. Physiol, 594(20), 5749-5768.

11 Khan Academy on https://www.khanacademy.org/test-prep/mcat/biological-sciences-practice/biological-sciences-practice-tut/e/innate-vs-adaptive-immunity

12Lleff, John. (2014) Searching for the Mind Blog. On http://jonlieffmd.com/blog/non-immune-cells-also-combat-microbes

13 Wiig, H., et al. (2010). Interaction between the extracellular matrix and lymphatics: consequences for lymphangiogenesis and lymphatic function. Matrix biology J.Internl. Soc Matrix Biology, 29(8), 645-56.

14 Naviaux, Robert, et al. (2016) Metabolic features of chronic fatigue syndrome. *Proc. Royal. Acad. Sciences*. May. https://www.pnas.org/content/pnas/early/2016/08/24/1607571113.full.pdf

15 Braden, Greg (2006). The Divine Matrix; Bridging Time, Space, Miracles and Belief. Hay House

16 Braden, Greg (2017) Human by Design: from Evolution by Chance, to Transformation by Choice. Hay House.

17Worby, P. (2018). The Scar that won't Heal. Createspace.

18 Pert, Candace. (1999). The Molecules of Emotion: Why You Feel the Way You Feel- Simon and Shuster

19Kormos V, Gaszner (2013). B. Role of neuropeptides in anxiety, stress, and depression: from animals to humans. Neuropeptides. Dec;47(6):401-19. doi: 10.1016/j.npep.2013.10.014.

20Goldsmith DR et al. (2016). A meta-analysis of blood cytokine network alterations in psychiatric patients: comparisons between schizophrenia, bipolar disorder and depression. Mol Psychiatry. Dec;21(12):1696-1709. doi: 10.1038/mp.2016.3. Epub 2016 Feb 23.

21CarnigliaL et al. (2017). Neuropeptides and Microglial Activation in Inflammation, Pain, and Neurodegenerative Diseases. Mediators Inflamm.;5048616. doi: 10.1155/2017/5048616.

22 Varshney P et al. (2016). Lipid rafts in immune signalling: current progress and future perspective. Immunology. Sep;149(1):13-24. doi: 10.1111/imm.12617.

23Davis TP. et al. (2015). Peptides at the blood brain barrier: Knowing me knowing you. Peptides. Oct;72:50-6. doi: 10.1016/j.peptides.2015.04.020.

24 Rieger, Berndt. Hashimoto's Healing. 2014. Self published (some in English) available on his website. www.Berndt-Rieger.de

25 William, Anthony (2017). Medical Medium Thyroid Healing: The Truth behind Hashimoto's, Graves', Insomnia, Hypothyroidism, Thyroid Nodules & Epstein-Barr. Hay House

26 ibid

27K Sri N. (2015). Mobile Phone Radiation: Physiological &Pathophysiologcal Considerations. Indian J. PhysiolPharmacol. Apr-Jun;59(2):125-35.

28 Zhou, L., & Foster, J. A. (2015). Psychobiotics and the gut–brain axis: in the pursuit of happiness. Neuropsychiatric Disease and Treatment, 11, 715–723. http://doi.org/10.2147/NDT.S61997.

29 Suez, et al. (2018). Post-Antibiotic Gut Mucosal Microbiome Reconstitution Is Impaired by Probiotics and Improved by Autologous FMT, Cell 174, 1406–1423. September 6-142 doi:h10.1016/j.cell.2018.08.0473.e16

30 Ennis, Cath. (2014). Epigenetics 101: a beginner's guide to explaining everything. The Guardian Science page. https://www.theguardian.com/science/occams-corner/2014/apr/25/epigenetics-beginners-guide-to-everything.

31 Bland, Jeffrey S (2014).. The Disease Delusion; Conquering the Causes of Chronic Illness for a Healthier, Longer, and Happier Life. Harper Collins

[32] Quoted by Dr Paul Beaver in Interpreting your genetics Summit April 2019. Own notes

33 Tips, Jack. The Cholesterol Myth: A Deception of Mammoth Proportions. Open Health Book.com. Pdf downloaded from AppleADayPressjack @wellnesswiz.com

34 Mercola, Joseph. Why Cholesterol is Essential for Optimal Health, and the Six Most Important Risk Factors of Heart Disease. http://articles.mercola.com/sites/ articles/ archive/2012/12/30/cholesterol-levels.aspx.

35 Lipton, Bruce. (2005). The Biology of Belief; Unleashing the power of consciousness, matter and miracles. Cygnus Books P172.

36 Bland, Jeffrey S (2014). The Disease Delusion; Conquering the Causes of Chronic Illness for a Healthier, Longer and Happier Life, Harper Wave, P242

37 Singh, V. P., et al. (2014). Advanced Glycation End Products and Diabetic Complications. Korean J. Physiol & Pharmacol. : 18(1), 1–14.

38 Gkogkolou, P., & Böhm, M. (2012). Advanced glycation end products: Key players in skin aging? Dermato-Endocrinology, 4(3), 259–270. http://doi.org/10.4161/derm.22028.

[39] Uribarri, J., et al. (2015). Dietary advanced glycation end products and their role in health and disease. *Advances in nutrition* (Bethesda, Md.), 6(4), 461-73. doi:10.3945/an.115.008433

40 San Gil, R., et al. (2017). The heat shock response in neurons and astroglia and its role in neurodegenerative diseases. Mol. neurodegeneration, 12(1), 65.

41 Xu, C. et al. (2014). Light-harvesting chlorophyll pigments enable mammalian mitochondria to capture photonic energy and produce ATP. J. Cell Sci. Jan 15;127(Pt 2):388-99.

42 Cameron, Tom (2017). Protomorphogens. Accessed at https://ivcjournal.com/protomorphogens/

43 ibid

44 Samsel, A., & Seneff, S. (2013). Glyphosate, pathways to modern diseases II: Celiac sprue and gluten intolerance. Interdisciplinary toxicology, 6(4), 159-84.

45 Samsel A, Seneff S (2016). Glyphosate pathways to modern diseases V: amino acid analogue of glycine in diverse proteins. J Biol Phys Chem 16:9–49.10.4024/03SA16A.jbpc.16.01

[46] Seneff, Stephanie.. (2018). How glyphosate poisoning explains the peculiarities of the autism gut. http://www.greenmedinfo.com/blog/how-glyphosate-poisoning-explains-peculiarities-autism-gut

47McCance and Widdowson (2016). data quoted in the Cytoplan manual. Cytoplan UK.

48 Pert, Candace. (1999). The Molecules of Emotion: Why You Feel the Way You Feel- Simon and Shuster P185

[49] ibid

50 Worby, P (2017). The World Within; how your microbiome makes you who you are. Kdp/ Createspace

51NHS pharmacists for NHS healthcare professionals. Should patients on statins take Coenzyme Q10 supplementation to reduce the risk of myotoxicity?www.medicinesresources.nhs.uk%2Fupload%2FNHSE_Co_enzyme_

Q_and_statins_46_4%2520Final%5B1%5D.doc

52 Cunha, JP. Medicine Net Accessed 2018. https://www.medicinenet.com/mercury_poisoning/article.htm#mercury_poisoning_definition_and_facts

53 Carnahan, Jill. (2015). Mold Testing Interview with High Intensity Health. Accessed on https://www.youtube.com/watch?v=4_8UOUsM_rY

54 Mercola, J. https://articles.mercola.com/sites/articles/archive/2008/06/21/are-you-allergic-to-wireless-internet.aspx Accessed on 20/2/19

55 Shakya, H, Christakis, N (2017) Association of Facebook Use With Compromised Well-Being: A Longitudinal Study, American Journal of Epidemiology, Volume 185, Issue 3, 1 February, Pages 203–211

56 Berryman C, et al (2018). Social Media Use and Mental Health among Young Adults..Psychiatr Q. Jun;89(2):307-314. doi: 10.1007/s11126-017-9535-6

[57] Brown, Daniel, (2015) The Attachment Project online training programme, www..attachmentproject.com accessed on 8.4.19

58 Le Doux, Joseph (1999) The Emotional Brain; The Mysterious Underpinnings of Emotional Life. W&N; New Ed edition (4 Feb. 1999

59 Goldstein D.S. et al. (2013). Determinants of buildup of the toxic dopamine metabolite DOPAL in Parkinson's disease. J Neurochem.126(5):591-603.

60 Naviaux R (2018) Metabolic features and regulation of the healing cycle—A new model for chronic disease pathogenesis and treatment. Mitochondrion

[61] DeMartini, John (2015) Just how valuable do you think you are? Downloaded from https://drdemartini.com/what-are-values/ on 18/1/19

[62] Hickie, Ian B. (2013) Manipulating the sleep-wake cycle and circadian rhythms to improve clinical management of major depression. *BMC Medicine* 11:79 https://doi.org/10.1186/1741-7015-11-79

[63] Dopico, X. C., et al. (2015). Widespread seasonal gene expression reveals annual differences in human immunity and physiology. Nature Communications, 6, 7000. http://doi.org/10.1038/ncomms8000.

[64] Hunt, S. J. & Navalta, J. W. (2012). Nitric Oxide and the Biological Cascades Underlying Increased Neurogenesis, Enhanced Learning Ability, and Academic Ability as an Effect of Increased Bouts of Physical Activity. International Journal of Exercise Science, 5(3), 245–275.

[65] He F, et al. (2016). Redox Mechanism of Reactive Oxygen Species in Exercise. Front Physiol. 2016 Nov 7;7:486.

[66] Belviranli, M, Okudan, N. Well-Known Antioxidants and Newcomers in Sport Nutrition: Coenzyme Q10, Quercetin, Resveratrol, Pterostilbene, Pycnogenol and Astaxanthin. Editors, In: Lamprecht M, (Ed) in Antioxidants in Sport Nutrition. Boca Raton (FL): CRC Press/Taylor & Francis; 2015. Chapter 5.

67 Cockcroft EJ et al. High intensity interval exercise is an effective alternative to moderate intensity exercise for improving glucose tolerance and insulin

sensitivity in adolescent boys. J Sci Med Sport. 2015 Nov;18(6):720-4.

68 Hollick, Michael. (2011). The Vitamin D solution. Plume

69 Samuel S1, Sitrin MD (2008) Vitamin D's role in cell proliferation and differentiation Nutr Rev. Oct;66(10 Suppl 2):S116-24. doi: 10.1111/j.1753-4887.2008.00094.x.

[70] Seneff, S., et al. (2015). A novel hypothesis for atherosclerosis as a cholesterol sulfate deficiency syndrome. *Theoretical biology & medical modelling, 12*, 9. doi:10.1186/s12976-015-0006-1

[71] Seneff, S. et al. (2015). A novel hypothesis for atherosclerosis as a cholesterol sulfate deficiency syndrome. Theor Biol Med Model. 2015; 12(1): 9).

72 Oschman, J. L., Chevalier, G., & Brown, R. (2015). The effects of grounding (earthing) on inflammation, the immune response, wound healing, and prevention and treatment of chronic inflammatory and autoimmune diseases. *J Inflamm Res*, 8, 83–96. http://doi.org/10.2147/JIR.S69656.

73Chevalier G, et al. (2012) Review article: Earthing: health implications of reconnecting the human body to the Earth's surface electrons. J Environ Public Health: 291541.

[74] Ober, Clint. (2014). Earthing. Basic Health Publications, Inc.; 2nd edition

[75] Pinault, Nick (2019). How 5G & EMF Radiation Impact Your Health. N & G Media Inc.

[76] https://www.theguardian.com/technology/2018/jul/14/mobile-phones-cancer-inconvenient-truths

[77] Pall M. L. (2013). Electromagnetic fields act via activation of voltage-gated calcium channels to produce beneficial or adverse effects. Journal of cellular and molecular medicine, 17(8), 958–965. doi:10.1111/jcmm.12088

[78] Pall M.L. (2018). Wi-Fi is an important threat to human health. *Environ Res.* Jul;164:405-416. doi: 10.1016/j.envres.2018.01.035. Epub 2018 Mar 21.

[79] Moon, Debbie. (2018). Autophagy Genes. In Genetic Life Hacks accessed on https://www.geneticlifehacks.com/autophagy-genes/ 1/2/19

[80] Tonelli, C., Chio, I., & Tuveson, D. A. (2018). Transcriptional Regulation by Nrf2. Antioxidants & redox signalling, 29(17), 1727-1745.

[81] Pompa, True Cellular Detox™ (2016), Revelation Health LLC.

[82] Harman D. The biologic clock: the mitochondria? *J Am Geriatr Soc.* 1972 Apr; 20(4):145-7.

[83] Kudryavtseva, A., et al. (2016). Mitochondrial dysfunction and oxidative stress in aging and cancer. *Oncotarget,* 7(29), 44879-44905.

[84] Bland, J. (2014). *The Disease Delusion*: Conquering the Causes of Chronic Illness for a Healthier, Longer, and Happier Life. Harper Wave. P280

[85] Lange, C. et al. (2016) Vascular endothelial growth factor: a neurovascular target in neurological diseases. Nature Reviews Neurology 12, 439–454

86 Longo, V. The Longevity Diet: Discover the New Science Behind Stem Cell Activation and Regeneration to Slow Aging, Fight Disease, and Optimize Weight. New York: Avery/Penguin Books, 2018

87 Golan, Ralph (1998). Optimal Wellness, Wellspring/Ballantine P228.

88 Wentz, Isabella (2017). Why women have more thyroid disorders Blog on https://thyroidpharmacist.com/articles/women-thyroid-disorders/

89 ibid

90 Rom, Aviva. (2106). Microbiome Summit May 2016. Personal notes

91 Smeyne, M., & Smeyne, R. J. (2013). Glutathione metabolism and Parkinson's disease. Free radical biology & medicine, 62, 13-25.

92 Pert, Candace (1998). Molecules of emotion P182

93 Kharrazian, Datis. (2017) Broken Brain film series transcript.

94 De la Monte, S. M., & Wands, J. R. (2008). Alzheimer's Disease Is Type 3 Diabetes–Evidence Reviewed. J. Diabetes Sci Tech, 2(6), 1101–1113.

95 Pan, W., et al. (2011). Cytokine signalling modulates blood-brain barrier function. Curr. pharma design, 17(33), 3729-40.

96 Rosales-Corral S. et a l. (2015) Diabetes and Alzheimer disease, two overlapping pathologies with the same background: oxidative stress. Oxid Med Cell Longev. 985845. doi: 10.1155/2015/985845. Epub 2015 Feb 26.

97 Saharan S, Mandal PK. The emerging role of glutathione in Alzheimer's disease. J. Alzheimers Dis. 2014;40(3):519-29. doi: 10.3233/JAD-132483.

98 Graff-Radford, J and Kantarci, K. (2013). Magnetic resonance spectroscopy in Alzheimer's disease. Neuropsychiatric Disease Treatment, 9, 687–696. http://doi.org/10.2147/NDT.S35440.

99 Bryan, T (2018). You Can Fix Your Brain: Just 1 Hour a Week to the Best Memory, Productivity, and Sleep You've Ever Had Rodale.

100 Lieff, J. (2014). Searching for the mind. They dynamic relationship of mitochondria and neurons. http://jonlieffmd.com/blog/dynamic-relationship-of-mitochondria-and-neurons Accessed 4.3.19

101 ibid

102 ibid

103 Genova, Lisa. (2017). TED talk. What you can do to prevent Alzheimers https://www.ted.com/talks/lisa_genova_what_you_can_do_to_prevent_alzheimer_s?language=en#t-159969. accessed on 7/2/19

104 Bredesen, Dale. (2017) The End of Alzheimer's: The First Programme to Prevent and Reverse the Cognitive Decline of Dementia. Vermillion.

105 Bredesen, Dale. Broken Brain Episode 3: Losing your Mind. Own notes.

106 Pasqualetti G. et al (2016). Cognitive Function and the Ageing Process: The Peculiar Role of Mild Thyroid Failure Endocr Metab Immune Drug Discov. 10(1):4-10.

107 Landel, V et al (2016). Vitamin D, Cognition and Alzheimer's Disease: The Therapeutic Benefit is in the D-Tails J. Alzheimer's Disease, 53(2):419-444,

108 Etgen T , Sander et al. (2012) Vitamin D deficiency, cognitive impairment and dementia: A systematic review and meta-analysis. Dement Geriatr Cogn Disord 33, 297–305.

109 Littlejohns TJ, Henley WE, Lang IA, et al. Vitamin D and the risk of dementia and Alzheimer disease. Neurology. 2014;83(10):920-928.

110 Miller JW., et al. (2015). Vitamin D Status and Rates of Cognitive Decline in a Multiethnic Cohort of Older Adults. JAMA Neurol. 72(11):1295–1303.

111 Soni M, Kos et al . (2012). Vitamin D and cognitive function. *Scand J Clin Lab Invest Suppl.* Apr;243:79-82.

112 Bronwell Logan (2013) The Overlooked Importance of Vitamin D Receptors Life Extension Magazine, August accessed on https://www.lifeextension.com/Magazine/2013/8/The-Overlooked-Importance-of-Vitamin-D-Receptors/Page-03

113 Hishikawa, N., et al. (2012). Effects of turmeric on Alzheimer's disease with behavioral and psychological symptoms of dementia. Ayu, 33(4), 499–504. http://doi.org/10.4103/0974-8520.110524.

[114] Galvin J. E. (2012). Optimizing Diagnosis and Management in mild to moderate Alzheimer's Disease. *Neurodegenerative disease management*, 2(3), 291–304. doi:10.2217/nmt.12.21

[115] Negandu, Tia et al (2015) A 2 year multidomain intervention of diet, exercise, cognitive training, and vascular risk monitoring versus control to prevent cognitive decline in at-risk elderly people (FINGER):a randomised controlled trial. The Lancet. http://dx.doi.org/10.1016/S0140-6736(15)60461-5

[116] Weikel, K. A., Chiu, C. J., & Taylor, A. (2012). Nutritional modulation of age-related macular degeneration. *Molecular aspects of medicine*, 33(4), 318–375. doi:10.1016/j.mam.2012.03.005

[117] ibid

118 Naviaux R.K. (2014). Metabolic features of the cell danger response. Mitochondrion: 16:7-17.

119 Naviaux R.K. (2016). Metabolic features of chronic fatigue syndrome. PNAS. 113; 37:472-480.

120 Xie, et al. (2013). Sleep drives metabolite clearance from the adult brain. Science. 18:342 373-7.

121 Alter H.J., et al. (2012). A multicenter blinded analysis indicates no association between chronic fatigue syndrome/myalgic encephalomyelitis and either xenotropic murine leukemia virus-related virus or polytropic murine leukemia virus. mBio 3(5):e00266-12.

122 Johnson, Cort. (2012). Lipkin Study Ends XMRV Saga: Lipkin Promises Progress on ME/CFS Pro Health magazine article accessed at http://www.prohealth.com/library/showarticle.cfm?libid=17220.

[123] Scott, Trudy (2011). The Anti-Anxiety Food solution New Harbinger.

[124] de la Fuente AG et al. Vitamin D receptor-retinoid X receptor heterodimer signalling regulates oligodendrocyte progenitor cell differentiation. J Cell Biol. 2015 Dec 7;211(5):975-85. doi: 10.1083/jcb.201505119.

[125] Wahls, Terry. Minding your Mitochondria TED talk. https://youtu.be/KLjgBLwH3Wc

126 The incidence and prevalence of Parkinson's in the UK. (2018). Clinical Research Practice Datalink. Accessed at https://www.parkinsons.org.uk/professionals/resources

127 Ahmed H., et al. (2017). Parkinson's disease and pesticides: A meta-analysis of disease connection and genetic alterations. Biomed Pharmacother. Jun;90:638-649. doi: 10.1016/j.biopha.2017.03.100. Epub 2017 Apr 14.

128 Breckenridge CB. Et al Association between Parkinson's Disease and Cigarette Smoking, Rural Living, Well-Water Consumption, Farming and Pesticide Use: Systematic Review and Meta-Analysis.PLoS One. 2016 Apr 7;11(4):e0151841. doi: 10.1371/journal.pone.0151841. eCollection 2016.

129 D'Errico, Get al. (2017). A current perspective on cancer immune therapy: step-by-step approach to constructing the magic bullet. Clin.transl. med, 6(1), 3.

130 Secombe KR et al (2018). The bidirectional interaction of the gut microbiome and the innate immune system: Implications for chemotherapy-induced gastrointestinal toxicity. Int J Cancer. Aug 28. doi: 10.1002/ijc.31836.

131 Servan-Schreiber, David (2011). Anti-Cancer: A new way of life. Michael Joseph.

132 Beliveaux, Richard (2017). Foods To Fight Cancer: What to Eat to Help Beat Cancer. Dorling Kindersley.

133 Hanahan D, and Weinberg RA (2011). Hallmarks of cancer: the next generation. Cell. Mar 4;144(5):646-74. doi: 10.1016/j.cell.2011.02.013.

134 Seyfried T. N. (2015). Cancer as a mitochondrial metabolic disease. Frontiers in cell and developmental biology, 3, 43. doi:10.3389/fcell.2015.00043

135 Tan et al., (2015). Mitochondrial genome acquisition restores respiratory function and tumourigenic potential of cancer cells without mitochondrial DNA. Cell Metab. 2015 Jan 6; 21(1):81-94.

136 Chinnery PF, Hudson G. Mitochondrial genetics. British medical bulletin. 2013;106:135–159

137 Christofferson, Travis (2017). Tripping over the Truth, Chelsea Green Publishing Co.

138 Winters, Nasha and Kelley, Jess. (2017). The Metabolic Approach to Cancer: Integrating Deep Nutrition, the Ketogenic Diet and Non-Toxic Bio-Individualized Therapies. Chelsea Green Publishing Co.

139 Calderon-Montano JM et al. (2011). Role of the Intracellular pH in the Metabolic Switch between Oxidative Phosphorylation and Aerobic Glycolysis - Relevance to Cancer. WebmedCentral, 2 (3), 1-10.hdl.handle.net/11441/53614

[140] Reshkin SJ et al. (2014). Role of pHi, and proton transporters in oncogene-driven neoplastic transformation. *Philos Trans R Soc Lond B Biol Sci.* Feb 3;369(1638):20130100. doi: 10.1098/rstb.2013.0100. Print 2014 Mar 19.

141 Damaghi Mehdi., et al. (2013). pH sensing and regulation in cancer Frontiers in Physiology Rev. 4 Dec: doi=10.3389/fphys.2013.00370

142 Schwartz L., et al (2017). Out of Warburg effect: An effective cancer treatment targeting the tumour specific metabolism and dysregulated pH. Semin Cancer Biol. Apr;43:134-138. doi: 10.1016/j.semcancer.2017.01.005.

[143] Cancer Research UK. Persistent Cancer Myths. https://scienceblog.cancerresearchuk.org/2014/03/24/dont-believe-the-hype-10-persistent-cancer-myths-debunked/#acidic-diets

144 Beliveau, Richard. (2017) Foods to Fight Cancer: What to Eat to Reduce your Risk. DK

[145] Servan-Schreiber. (2017) Anti-Cancer: a new way of Life. Penguin

146 Amin, A., et al. (2015). Sustained proliferation in cancer: Mechanisms and novel therapeutic targets. Seminars in cancer biology, 35 Suppl(Suppl), S25-S54.

147 Jafri, M. A et al. (2016). Roles of telomeres and telomerase in cancer, and advances in telomerase-targeted therapies. Genome medicine, 8(1), 69. doi:10.1186/s13073-016-0324-x

[148] Medicinal Mushrooms PDQ (2017). NIH National Cancer Institute. Accessed https://www.cancer.gov/about-cancer/treatment/cam/patient/mushrooms-pdq

149 Parks SK., et al (2017). Hypoxia and cellular metabolism in tumour pathophysiology. J Physiol. Apr 15;595(8):2439-2450. doi: 10.1113/JP273309

[150] Duan C. (. 2016) Hypoxia-inducible factor 3 biology: complexities and emerging themes. *Am J Physiol Cell Physiol* Feb 15;310(4):C260-9. doi: 10.1152/ajpcell.00315.2015. Epub 2015 Nov 11.

[151] Moritz, Andreas (2008) Cancer is not a disease it's a survival mechanism. Ener-chi.com.

[152] Paduch R. (2016). The role of lymphangiogenesis and angiogenesis in tumour metastasis. Cellular oncology (Dordrecht), 39(5), 397–410. doi:10.1007/s13402-016-0281-9

[153] Dawood S et al. (2014). Cancer stem cells: implications for cancer therapy. *Oncology* (Williston Park). Dec;28(12):1101-7, 1110.

[154] Longo, Valter. (2018).The Longevity Diet. Penguin Random House P36

[155] Ibid P 124

[156] Brandhorst, S. et al. (2015). A Periodic Diet that Mimics Fasting Promotes Multi-System Regeneration, Enhanced Cognitive Performance, and Healthspan. Cell metabolism, 22(1), 86-99.

[157] Seneff, Stephanie. (2012). Is Endothelial Nitric Oxide Synthase a Moonlighting

Protein Whose Day Job is Cholesterol Sulfate Synthesis? Implications for Cholesterol Transport, Diabetes and Cardiovascular Disease Entropy, 14(12), 2492-2530; doi:10.3390/e14122492 Review

[158] Wikipedia https://en.wikipedia.org/wiki/Ontogeny

[159] Achacoso, Ted. Human Longevity film Session 5: Sleep, Light and Disease. Own notes.

[160] HeartMath Institute. Study Shows Geomagnetic Fields and Solar Activity Affect Human Autonomic Nervous System Functions accessed https://www.heartmath.org/articles-of-the-heart/study-new-analysis-technique-support-group-synchronization-magnetic-fields/

[161] Schlitz M. (2016). The Grateful Aging Program: A Naturalistic Model of Transformation and Healing into the Second Half of Life. *The Permanente journal*, *21*, 16–082. doi:10.7812/TPP/16-082

162 Porges, Stephen. (2017). The Transforming Power of Feeling Safe. Workshop delivered for the Breath of Life Conference May 2017 Personal notes.

163 Laszlo, Ervin (2004). Science and the Akashic Field. An integral theory of everything. Inner Traditions.

[164] Burke-Harris, Nadine. TED talk. How childhood Health affects health outcomes. Accessed on https://www.ted.com/talks/nadine_burke_harris_how_childhood_trauma_affects_health_across_a_lifetime

[165] Radin, Dean. https://www.theepochtimes.com/supernormal-abilities-developed-through-meditation-dr-dean-radin-discusses_2157904.html

[166] ibid

[167] Ji, Sungchul (2018). The Cell Language Theory: Connecting Mind And Matter. World Scientific Europe

[168] Winkelmann S et al. (2006). The positive aspects of stress: strain initiates domain decondensation (SIDD).Brief Funct Genomic Proteomic. Mar;5(1):24-31.

[169] Liu, Richard T.; Alloy, Lauren B. (2010). "Stress generation in depression: A systematic review of the empirical literature and recommendations for future study". Clinical Psychology Review. 30 (5): 582–593.

170 Bland, Jeffrey S. (2016) in the Healthy Gut Summit January. Personal notes.

INDEX

45385898R00132

Printed in Poland
by Amazon Fulfillment
Poland Sp. z o.o., Wrocław